Quality Assurance for Biopharmaceuticals

Quality Assurance for Biopharmaceuticals

JEAN F. HUXSOLL

Matrix Pharmaceutical, Inc.

A Wiley-Interscience Publication

JOHN WILEY & SONS, INC.

New York / Chichester / Brisbane / Toronto / Singapore

Library of Congress Cataloging-in-Publication Data:

Huxsoll, Jean F.
     Quality assurance for biopharmaceuticals / Jean F. Huxsoll.
       p. cm.
     "A Wiley-Interscience publication".
     Includes bibliographical references and index.
     ISBN 0-471-03656-0
     1. Pharmaceutical biotechnology—Quality control. I. Title.
RS380.H88 1994
615'.19—dc20   93-46160
                                 CIP

Printed in the United States of America

10 9 8 7 6 5 4 3 2 1

Preface

The manufacture of biopharmaceuticals by biotechnological means is advancing and progressing rapidly. There are a large number of products with a variety of indications presently on the market. The list of products and indications will continue to grow over the next few years.

Since this industry is in its infancy, many facets are just starting to grow and develop. A few companies are in the adult stage, but the majority are still children. The intent of this book is to give some basic guidelines regarding quality assurance and its responsibilities for biopharmaceuticals manufactured by either recombinant, monoclonal antibody or other biotechnological methodologies. The topics were selected to give an introduction with some basic concepts of the quality assurance function. If the reader is interested in more in-depth information, the references at the end of each chapter will be a starting point.

The authors of each chapter are presently working in the biotechnology industry or recently were involved with the industry. Each author presents both the theoretical and practical aspects of the particular area discussed. It is very important to have this hands-on experience when giving guidance and input to the quality assurance function.

I want to thank each author for his or her time and efforts. Each was willing to share ideas and thoughts while continuing to work at a full-time job. I believe that the insight and suggestions given will be extremely worthwhile to both those individuals starting a quality assurance function and those already working in a quality assurance organization.

Special appreciation must be given for Barbara Miller, my Bay Area quality assurance colleague from James River Corporation, who sparked the first life into this book project, and without whose initiative the job might never have been completed.

I would also like to give a special thanks to Joel Torrevillas, Nicola Macfarlane, and Elaine Andrews for their efforts in organizing and word processing the chapters for this book.

The responsibilities and challenges of quality assurance are exciting and rewarding. I hope that those who read this book will benefit from the expertise and suggestions given and will be able to lead their industries in order to assure the safety, purity, and efficacy of the products produced.

Jean F. Huxsoll

Contents

Contributors

Frances M. Bogdansky, Director, Bioanalytical and Technical Services, Schering-Plough Research Institute, Kenilworth, NJ 07033

Charles Brochard, Director, Quality Assurance, Berlex Biosciences, Inc., 15049 San Pablo Ave., Richmond, CA 94804

Daniel R. Colton, Validation Engineer, Validation Engineering, Genentech, Inc., 460 Point San Bruno Blvd., South San Francisco, CA 94080

Elias L. Greene, Miles Inc., Fourth & Parker St., Berkeley, CA 94710

Jean F. Huxsoll, Vice President, Operations, Matrix Pharmaceutical, Inc., 1430 O'Brien Dr., Menlo Park, CA 94025

Don H. Miller, Materials Safety Manager, Quality Assurance, Miles Inc., Fourth & Parker St., Berkeley, CA 94710

Dorine Mulder, Director, Regulatory Affairs, EuroCetus B.V., Paasheuvelweg 30, 1105 BJ Amsterdam-Zuidoost, The Netherlands

Carolyn M. Orelli, Manager, GMP Compliance, Berlex Biosciences, Inc., 15049 San Pablo Ave., Richmond, CA 94804

Ralph H. Rousell, Miles Inc., Fourth & Parker St., Berkeley, CA 94710

Mary Sigourney, Manager, Regulatory Compliance, Microgenics Corporation, 2380A Bisso Ln., Concord, CA 94520

Cynthia L. Spencer, Attorney at Law, 1307 S. Mary Ave., Suite 209, Sunnyvale, CA 94087

Greg R. Swartz, Statistical Consultant, 303 Mariposa Ave., Mountain View, CA 94041

Ruth Wikberg-Leonardi, Associate Director, Regulatory Affairs, Gensia Pharmaceuticals, 1102 Roselle, San Diego, CA 92121

1 Organization of quality assurance

Jean F. Huxsoll

Contents

1.1 The quality function

1.1.1 The basic quality principles

Quality has many connotations. The companywide culture involves a total company commitment and philosophy. The term "total quality management" (TQM) is given to an approach that relates to the functioning of the company and the approach that "the company" uses to run day to day, develop, and improve. The philosophy of the Malcolm Baldridge National Quality Award (MBNQA) is based upon a company culture involving seven major categories: leadership, information and analysis, strategic quality planning, human resource development and management, management of process quality, quality and operational results, and customer focus and satisfaction. This book is not intended to describe a total company culture but is related to the specifics involved in the quality function of a biopharmaceutical company. Ideally, a company would develop both the culture and the function activities described in this book. Although not expressed in the specific terms, you will see many of these TQM philosophic aspects in the systems and approaches given in each chapter. As you read the various chapters you will recognize various parts of this TQM or MBNQA culture. Of prime importance is the customer and the ability to routinely use the complicated biotechnological production methods to produce products that will consistently yield the desired results.

This chapter is concerned with the organization of a unit of function within the company which has primary responsibility for quality assurance. It is intended to show how to establish and develop this unit. It in no way is meant to indicate that this function can replace TQM. This unit is part of the whole.

The principles of biotechnology are not new. The food industry is the oldest biotechnology industry. The manufacture of vinegar, alcoholic beverages, cheese, and sourdough are basic biotechnology processes, although it took years to understand their principles [1]. During World War I, acetone and glycerol were produced by biotechnology methods, and during World War II this methodology was used for large-scale fermentation of therapeutic antibiotics, including streptomycin and penicillin [2]. It generally has been accepted that a quality function is needed and required in food, drug, and cosmetic industries. The U.S. Code of Federal Regulations (CFR) defines the responsibilities of a quality control unit: It shall have the responsibility and authority to approve and reject all components, containers/closures, in-process materials, packaging materials, labeling, and drug products. The unit shall have responsibility and authority for approving or rejecting all procedures or specifications impacting on the strength, quality, and purity of any drug product. The total area of responsibility must be in writing [3]. This CFR-defined quality assurance (QA) organization is typical for a large majority of industries, not just food, drug, and cosmetic. The development of QA and its role has been slow. The necessity to mandate the role of QA in the CFR supports this. The U.S. government defines the quality unit, and industry is obligated to follow the mandate. In many companies, particularly small, start-up companies, QA is looked upon as overhead; the unit does not function, or is not allowed to function, as part of the company team, and neither the company nor the unit understands the role and responsibilities of the QA unit.

The development of the biotechnology, or "biotech", industry for biopharmaceuticals is exciting and rapid. Many new, small companies have been, or are being, established. The main emphasis of these companies is the development of the science associated with their particular products. There is a tendency to develop the science and leave the quality function in the background. For the ultimate success of the company, it is important to start developing the QA function in parallel with the science.

In larger, established companies, the role and responsibilities of QA is understood. There is usually no need to establish the worth and need of the function. But, in the experience of the author, there is little understanding regarding the need or purpose of the quality function in small, start-up companies. Parts of this introductory chapter will be aimed at these small companies, although the concepts are not so limited. The contents of the book cover all areas relating to quality and will be references for the quality function, no matter the size of the company or the size of the department.

The first QA activity usually undertaken in the biopharmaceutical environment is the quality control (QC) function, which is primarily a testing function. Test methods are developed to give an indication of the product consistency and identity. In many instances at these early stages, methods are developed but no QA activities are undertaken to assure the meaningfulness of the assays and their reproducibility. New companies are aware that they need some sort of quality function, and a QC unit is started and given the primary responsibility for performing QC testing. This unit often reports to research and development (R&D). QC in this sense is extremely limited and in no way encompasses the total scope of the quality responsibility. Many such companies do not even realize their lack of comprehensive QA functions and systems.

It is clear that, although the biopharmaceutical industry is in its infancy, the requirements for QA are no different for this industry than for other industries. In biotech, QA encompasses a broader range of items, such as clinical studies (as reflected in the GLPs) and product consistency. QA is a necessary function that must be integrated into the company at an early stage of its development. The old standby definitions of initial experts in the field are still very appropriate for the biotechnology industry. Dr. Joseph Juran defines quality as "fitness for use" [4]. Figure 1.1 illustrates this definition.

There are four major components of his fitness for use:
1. quality of design,
2. quality of conformance,
3. availability, and
4. field service.

These four major categories are further subdivided; the twelve subdivisions are necessary no matter what the manner of manufacture or the product being manufactured:
1. quality of market research,
2. quality of concept,
3. quality of specification,
4. technology,
5. manpower,
6. management,
7. reliability,
8. maintainability,
9. logistical support,
10. promptness,
11. competence, and
12. integrity.

Also, for the biopharmaceutical industry, conformance to regulatory standards is a requirement.

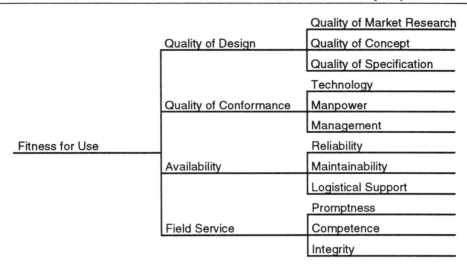

Figure 1.1 "Fitness for use" components

Source: J.M. Juran, Quality Control Handbook, 3d edition, McGraw-Hill, Inc., 1974. This material is reproduced with permission of McGraw-Hill, Inc.

Dr. W. Deming has a fourteen-point top management plan for quality. Again, as with Dr. Juran, these points are valid for any industry. The main emphasis of his fourteen points is to have the commitment and the involvement of upper management in a quality plan. Mass inspection should be eliminated, and statistical methods should be instituted and used. Training and two-way communication should be established. Due to the complexity of biopharmaceutical products, "quality of manufacture" becomes critical and is the main means of assuring consistency and acceptability.

Dr. A.V. Feigenbaum defines QA as "an effective system for integrating the quality-development, quality-maintenance, and quality-improvement efforts of various groups in an organization so as to enable marketing, engineering, production, and service at the most economical levels which allow for full customer satisfaction" [5].

The CFR has included a definition of the QA unit under the section for good laboratory practice (GLP) [6]. There are seven points:

1. Maintain a copy of the master schedule sheet of all nonclinical laboratory studies.
2. Maintain copies of all protocols pertaining to all nonclinical laboratory studies.
3. Inspect each phase of a nonclinical laboratory study.
4. Periodically submit written status reports.
5. Determine that no deviations from approved protocols or standard operating procedure (SOP) were made without proper authorization and documentation.
6. Review the final study report to assure that such report accurately describes the methods and SOP.
7. Prepare and sign a statement to be included with the final study report which shall specify the dates inspections were made and findings reported to management.

It is important for QA to develop both the necessary expertise and systems early on to help support the company as it grows. To function effectively in this GLP role in the biopharmaceutical area, the QA function must understand the purpose and extent of the clinical studies.

1.1.2 QC versus QA

One of the greatest points of confusion regarding the quality function is the difference between QC and QA. QC is a very limited function that "controls" the product, primarily by testing. This concept goes back to the old definition of quality as a police function with the idea that the quality can be tested into a product. Unfortunately, too many "start-up" biotechnology companies are operating in this mode. QC is established to test the product. Although the CFR uses the term "quality control", their definition is, in reality, more a definition of QA. The GLPs try to give some meaning to the definition, and they use the term "quality assurance". This definition is in no way complete.

QA is the function that sets up the systems and methods for "assuring" the quality of the product. The product is defined by the methods of manufacture, not by the end test results. This is commonly referred to as "building the quality into the product". R.R. Pedraja refers to the "Quality Spectrum". This is the quality of people, quality of communications, quality of environment, quality of systems, quality of services, quality of technology, and quality of products [7].

The intent of this book is to present a general guideline to the QA function and its various aspects that are related to the biotechnology industry. In some cases, these responsibilities and functions will not be different from those in any other industry; in some cases, they will be more involved or will carry a different emphasis. All of the authors recently have had involvement, or are presently involved, in some aspect of the quality function as it relates to the biotechnology industry. An attempt is made to present some hands-on experiences and recommendations.

1.2 Responsibilities of quality functions

1.2.1 Routine functions

There are a number of routine quality functions that are necessary for all industries:
1. testing,
2. documentation,
3. labeling,
4. vendor audits,
5. vendor approval,
6. raw material receipt,
7. product release
8. product specifications
9. training, and
10. validation.

Testing of raw materials, in-process materials, and final product will be covered in detail in later chapters. Documentation of a variety of activities, including QA/QC procedures, assay validation, facility validation, process validation, manufacturing records, and complaints will be discussed throughout the book. Labeling responsibilities include the development of the labeling, the approval of the master labeling, the issuance of the correct labels, and the verification that the correct label was used. A large percentage of recalls are due to labeling errors. Although this appears to be a relatively easy function, it must be performed by trained individuals, and resources must be provided to correctly perform the function. Presently regulations, or guidelines, are being developed as part of the GMPs for labeling. Vendor audits and vendor approval are keys to building acceptable product. These functions are recognized in older industries but may be ignored in young biotech. It is important to address these functions early in the process development. QA does not necessarily have total responsibility for these but should assure that they are addressed.

Raw material receipt by the quality function, with inspection and testing, is necessary. Product release is one of the more obvious functions that is not generally overlooked. Product specifications must be reviewed and approved by the quality function. Training and validation are necessary components of the function. Again, these are functions that may be overlooked in start-up situations. Validation is best placed in that function that has the greatest knowledge of the activity. It is not mandated that it be in QA, but QA should have both an approval and audit responsibility.

1.2.2 Necessary but not obvious functions

There are a few areas important to the success of the quality function that are necessary but, in some cases, not obvious:

1. company awareness,
2. product knowledge,
3. facility knowledge,
4. networking through outside organizations, and
5. risk analysis/decision making.

Company awareness regards both long- and short-term goals and objectives. The quality function should be part of the team that develops the company business plan. The quality function should not operate as a separate entity, and it should understand the future of the company. The total management of the company must commit to this approach and understanding. Product knowledge is critical to the success of the quality function. The quality organization must understand the product, process, support systems, and product use. Without this expertise, the group will operate in a vacuum and will not be able to establish the necessary systems. As will be discussed throughout this book, the product must be defined by the systems that are established to assure its consistency.

Facility knowledge is also extremely important to the successful operation of this function. Many of the controlled parameters of the process depend upon the functions of the equipment and facility. Without expertise in this area, the quality team will not be able to participate as part of the working organization. There is a tendency to operate and make decisions and establish systems independent of other operations. In the opinion of the author, it is absolutely impossible for a quality function to operate without both product and facility expertise.

The processes of biotechnology are complicated and offer many alternatives for interpretation. Networking through outside organizations yields resources both to further educate oneself and to acquire expertise and exposure to areas outside the company. It may be critical to establishing systems within one's own company to understand regulatory and industry systems standards that have been developed and established.

Last, but by no means least, is risk analysis/decision making. The expertise and knowledge that the other areas give the quality function help to establish the ability for this most critical aspect of the function. Obviously, there is a need to guarantee the safety, purity, and efficacy of the product. The ability to analyze the situations and make recommendations may be the most meaningful of the quality functions.

1.2.3 Industry quality functions

Although it may seem obvious that quality systems are necessary, many small or start-up companies function, or try to function, with only some areas covered. A survey performed in 1988 indicates the breadth of the systems established within the industry. Table 1.1 summarizes the systems and the percentages of the companies responding to the survey that had established these systems. The age of the company and the industry had some effect on the extensiveness of the quality function activities [8]. It is clear that testing is the primary emphasis. This supports

Table 1.1   Percentages of companies responding to 1988 survey reporting establishment of quality systems

Quality Functions	System Established (%)
Final Product Testing	82.1
Final Product Release	78.0
In-Process Testing	74.0
Raw Material Testing	69.9
Establish Specifications	69.9
Approve Specifications	69.9
Label Control	66.7
Raw Material Release	62.6
Approve Labeling	60.2
Approve Process Documents	59.3
Assay Development	56.9
Equipment Validation	56.1
In-Process Release	54.5
Vendor Approval	52.8
Statistical Sampling	52.9
Disposition Non-conforming Material	52.0
Process Validation	46.3
Vendor Audits	35.0
Trend Charting	30.9
Vendor Surveillance	26.8
Control Charting	24.4
Statistical Process Control	16.3

Source: J. Huxsoll, et al.; *Regulatory Affairs*, 2 (1990):299-318.

the observation that testing or QC is perceived, at least in the beginning, as the emphasis of the quality function.

It is interesting to note that most of these functions are part of the GMPs, and most individuals responding to the survey felt biotechnology companies were obligated to follow the GMPs, although less than 50% of them were using half of the systems listed. The intent of the GMPs is to establish the necessary quality systems that assure the building in of quality during processing, rather than the testing of quality at the end.

1.3 Establishing an organization

1.3.1 Define QA function

Most QA functions in biotechnology companies will be established while the company is small. Ideally, the function should be developed prior to starting production of Phase I clinical material. A key in the success of these companies will be developing systems early that will support and benefit the product and the company.

At the onset, there should be a conscious decision to define and establish what quality systems are necessary. Most companies will not have the luxury to start out with a large group of individuals to carry on all potential activities. It will be necessary to determine which functions are necessary and important for their particular situation and for QA to detail for company management any risks involved with deleting any of these functions.

When defining the functions, it should be determined what the company can, should, and desires to accomplish. The type of product, the production method, the complexity of the end material, and the stage of development will be key to the decisions. In the original assessment, the key to making the right decisions is consideration of the end use of the product and the necessity to assure its purity, safety, and potential efficacy. There will undoubtedly be financial constraints. This will make the initial analysis more difficult and make it extremely important that the right systems be established.

As a side note on the initial recommendation, it is likely that some managers of other departments who must "buy into" the plan will not totally understand the need for QA functions. Explanations and recommendations will be required. This first step is critical to the long-term success of the total company. The plan and organization should be documented in writing. The analysis should involve the total company and should emphasize a long-term plan of development.

According to D. Hoernschemeyer, there are twelve facets to quality [9]:

1. Attitude that quality becomes a way of life,
2. Innovation that everyone is involved in quality,
3. Integrity where quality indicators are discussed rather than hidden,
4. Information so that everyone understands goals and policies and so there is feedback concerning results,
5. Support where people are encouraged and accomplishments are recognized,
6. Resources in regard to both time and people,
7. Dialogue that is continuous between departments,
8. Relationships that erase the police image,
9. Goals and plans as are necessary for any activity,
10. Long-term view is established for quality improvements avoiding the necessity to have firefighting activities,

11. Embracing change for all activities to improve, and
12. Offering no myths or excuses for failures.

To the quality professional, these activities and thoughts seem second nature, but they are not as easy to establish and carry out as one would like. Biotechnology brings another facet to the quality function due to the complexity of the product and the process required to make the product.

1.3.1.1 Examples of QA functions

The average start-up organization will not be able to conduct all of these functions. Based upon the experience of the author, certain functions are necessary for the initial start-up as the core of the organization. The other activities can grow as the company and quality organization grow.

The QA group may have responsibility but must have approval authority with audit capabilities for the following areas:
1. assay development and validation,
2. equipment validation,
3. process validation,
4. vendor qualifications,
5. raw material and product specifications,
6. documentation, and
7. QC testing.

The primary responsibility for these functions in small companies best resides in the function that has the greatest expertise. It is important for QA to become knowledgeable about these activities to give meaningful input. The QA approval must be accomplished in a manner that adds to the quality of the functions, rather than acting as an arbitrary veto power.

1.3.2 Define personnel requirements

Company management must support the quality plan. The most difficult aspect of the plan is its implementation. Two needs that must be addressed in the plan are: 1) the necessity to have the in-house product and facility expertise and 2) the need for out-of-house quality expertise. The advantages and disadvantages of in-house vs. out-of-house expertise for each function must be weighed, since it is important to avoid overstaffing in the beginning. Start out with minimal staff and add as a need arises. If QA is overstaffed in the beginning, the usefulness of some functions will not be totally recognized, and there will be continuing management pressure to cut back the QA function. A great key to success is to remember that others outside the quality organization should be a part of the everyday, ongoing QA activities. If the total organization understands the necessity of the QA goals and actions, this is not a difficult task; therefore, it is important to have a strong program to educate the total company about the quality function and quality responsibilities.

Too many times, the role of the QA organization is not understood, and the quality function is looked upon as unnecessary overhead. This attitude can and must be avoided. In some instances, the QA personnel will have to earn the respect and understanding of the staff from other areas. QA may need to learn both the equipment and processes to accomplish this respect. The ability of QA to become part of the team, with a company commitment and understanding, will be critical to the success of the company.

The initial quality team should have some product expertise, but it must also have quality expertise. For example, someone who has worked in R&D cannot move directly into QA and set up the quality functions without prior QA experience or knowledge. The individual leading the QA group must hold a high enough management position so that he or she may interact with personnel from other functions within the company and have the authority to make substantial decisions. This person must have a strong background in quality activities and needs to have "people skills" so that there will be successful communication with other departments in the company. Quality must function as part of the team to be successful.

1.3.2.1 Examples of QA organizations

The following organization charts are some examples of starting organizations. A minimal staff must cover documentation, testing, process validation/control support, and vendor acceptability. Each of these functions takes someone experienced in the area covered. An ideal start-up organization should include documentation; testing, including stability; validation of equipment, processes, and assays; and a systems group for establishing specifications, setting up systems, releasing product, and handling discrepancies and complaints.

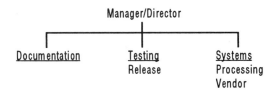

Figure 1.2 Organization with minimal staff

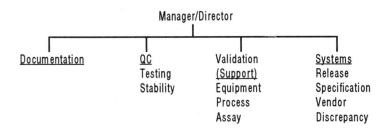

Figure 1.3 Organization for start-up company

1. 4   Day-to-day operations

1.4.1   Setting standards

Once goals and objectives for the company have been established, the quality function must set standards within these objectives for both its own activities and those of the company. These standards must be in writing. Standards are necessary for vendors, raw materials, documentation, in-process testing and inspection, validation, and final product specifications. Standards are necessary for process and testing deviations and for the overall activities of the company. If meaningful standards are established that are supported, carrying out this activity becomes easy. On the other hand, if the quality function does not have the necessary leadership and expertise, either setting up or carrying out these standards becomes extremely difficult.

Daily standards must be based upon expectations and experience with the end product. It is necessary to know the difference between minor and major issues. This is a critical item for biopharmaceuticals when the process is critical to defining the product. This distinction is difficult and sometimes erodes the credibility of the quality function, especially when their scientific background is weak. It is much easier to support the stand that everything is black and white; in reality, most issues are gray. The key is the ability to analyze and understand all aspects of the situation.

1.4.2   Implementing training

Training and the development of individuals in all functions is important to conduct on a daily basis. The individuals in the quality function also must be given the opportunity and time for adequate training. For QA to function in a meaningful capacity, the training must include various areas of the manufacturing process as well as the standard quality functions. Each individual must be given adequate time and support, and the training program must have the financial backing of the organization.

As with all production environments, the activities of the quality function encompasses a significant amount of time and effort. It is necessary to make formal plans for the time and types of training to be given. If this is not done, other activities will take precedence and, as a result, there will be little or no training. One means of accomplishing formal training is to add the specifics of the training into an individual's goals and objectives for the year. This gives the individual and his or her supervisor the impetus to follow up and to push for the training. It is also helpful to set aside specific times during the day or week for the training. It may even be possible to set up internships so that individuals from different departments trade work functions. QA also has a responsibility to audit the training records of all company functions.

1.4.3   Realistic feedback

To establish effective and meaningful systems, the company needs to understand and appreciate what is being implemented and accomplished by the quality function. A system for realistic feedback is needed. Feedback has to be both positive and negative if it is going to be helpful. In a biotechnology atmosphere where the processes are ongoing for many days at a time, the end product's quality is defined by the process, and it is absolutely necessary to have timely, realistic feedback. It may be necessary to make decisions during the process rather than at the end, when releasing the product.

1.4.4   Follow-through

Along with feedback, it is necessary to have follow through. If commitments are made, they must be completed unless there is some extenuating circumstance. As with any manufacturing activity, communication becomes a key to the success of this activity. It is necessary to set up systems and personnel that can handle the activity. If QA support is needed, then it is important that the activity be handled in a timely manner. If decisions and activities happen without QA support, the tendency will be to continue without this support, and it will appear to most that the quality function is not necessary.

The quality function must understand and support time commitments and constraints of other activities. The quality function has an obligation and responsibility to function within the same time constraints as the rest of the company. Activities must be carried out to fruition.

1.5 Conclusion

The traditional definitions of QA are appropriate for the biotechnology industry. The standard systems and methodologies become the core for the function. The organization must understand not only the role of the QA function but the responsibilities of the organization toward product quality. The QA function establishes the systems, but everyone has a responsibility for quality. Quality must begin in the R&D area. QA must understand its role and how it relates to the mission of the company. The ongoing process of the biotechnology manufacturing atmosphere makes it important to define the product by the process. QA must take a positive, active role in this definition. There is absolutely no other way to guarantee the end product "fitness for use".

According to Hoernschemeyer, quality efforts fail for five reasons [8]. Three of these are specifically related to new start-up companies:

1. Vague or inaccurate perceptions of what quality means,
2. Lack of solid commitment and backing by top management, and
3. Belief by executives that a high level of quality can be achieved with a few techniques and devices. Added to this would be an additional belief that quality can be achieved by testing.

The role of QA in the biotechnology industry is complicated by the process methodology and the need to define the product by the process. The systems and the support activities are the key elements to this definition. The validation of all aspects of the process becomes the QA of the material. The means for determining the safety, efficacy, purity, and stability of the end material are related to this process definition.

This book is intended to give both general and specific information and guidelines to help establish, develop, and implement QA in a biopharmaceutical manufacturing environment.

References

[1] Knorr, D. and Sinskey, A.T. *Science 229* (1985):1224–1229.
[2] Pramer, D. *Bio/Technology 1* (1983):211–212.
[3] Title 21, Code of Federal Regulations, Section 200–209. Washington, DC: Office of the Federal Register, National Archives and Records Administration, 1989.
[4] Juran, J.M. *Quality Control Handbook,* 3d ed. New York: McGraw-Hill, 1974.
[5] Feigenbaum, A.U. *Total Quality Control.* New York: McGraw-Hill, 1983.
[6] Title 21, Code of Federal Regulations, Section 58.35. Washington, DC: Office of the Federal Register, National Archives and Records Administration, 1989.
[7] Pedraja, R.R. "Role of Quality Assurance in the Food Industry: New Concepts." *Food Technology* (Dec. 1988):92–93.
[8] Hoernschemeyer, D. "The Four Cornerstones of Excellence." *Quality Progress* (1989):38–40.

2 Coming into good manufacturing practice (GMP) compliance

C. M. Orelli

Contents

2.1   Profile of a research & development (Pre-GMP) company

There are several characteristics that most research and development (R&D) companies have in common. They generally start small, employing only a few people, and grow gradually to a few dozen employees. Initially, the majority of the employees are research scientists with a small number of production, testing, support, and administrative personnel.

This personnel profile results in some interesting situations at these small R&D companies. The personnel generally develop a company pride or operating style. Most often, this style, whether consciously or unconsciously, is different from the "corporate culture" found in large, established pharmaceutical companies. The R&D style is usually characterized by creativity and speed in answering challenges and solving problems. Due to the small size of the company, the personnel are able to react immediately to new situations or changing priorities. They are able to alter the direction of their research, and even their company, very quickly. Unfortunately for later retrieval and review, the communication (i.e., the decisions, background history, conclusions reached, etc.) is frequently only verbal, with no record of who decided what, when, and why. Operating in this fashion does allow the small company a very quick response time and speeds up the product development process, but there are some disadvantages. Key steps, decisions, process variations, and calculations may not be documented anywhere, and their eventual documentation may be difficult, or even impossible, to reconstruct. Process variations may produce a slightly different final product, cloud release issues, or even compromise studies such as long-term stability. This off-the-cuff operational style, if not monitored carefully and eventually modified, becomes an increasingly serious and costly liability as the company grows and the product gets closer to market.

2.2   Profile of a production (GMP compliant) company

Large, well-established pharmaceutical companies (i.e., those producing under GMP conditions) generally have several characteristics in common. These companies employ a larger number of individuals than R&D firms. The nature of the work usually requires that many personnel be concentrated in production, testing, support, and administrative functions. These personnel equal or outnumber (by as much as a factor of two) the research scientists. Due to the requirements and restrictions enforced by GMP compliance, the manufacturing and support personnel are not permitted to develop off-the-cuff solutions to challenges, but must follow accepted, validated, approved methods and secure predetermined approvals for changes or modifications. These constraints mean that changes usually cannot be implemented immediately, nor can direction be changed rapidly, even if situations or priorities suggest so. GMP regulations require documentation of actions, investigations, decisions and review (sometimes by a formal validation protocol), data collection and analysis, and reporting. As a result, communication is more formal and usually written.

2.3   How can a successful pre-GMP become a successful GMP compliant company?

2.3.1   Developing the plan

Once a pre-GMP company identifies a potential product, the first major task is to develop a plan or strategy to produce that product under GMP compliance. It is important that both the product and the plan conform to the overall master plan of the company. If the company has existing products, the new product should complement or be consistent with these. The product and development plan should be consistent with the company's established business strategy. If the product is not compatible with the facilities and equipment available on site, the plan must include provisions to modify buildings and equipment or to secure and validate production at another facility. This master plan will determine the breadth but not the intensity of the compliance activities required.

To develop a realistic plan with a realistic budget and time table, it is necessary to have personnel with regulatory experience. These people can be employees or consultants. In either case, it is important that they are experienced enough to guide the plan's development and to avoid unnecessary delays and costly mistakes [1].

Many people from different functions will be involved in achieving product and process compliance. It is important that these people have an understanding of the GMP regulations. While this knowledge can be gained by reading the regulations, it is more efficient to organize a group seminar. The presentation should include the history of the regulations, the reasons behind them, and the risks of failure to comply, as well as the benefits of compliance. Once the reasons and logic of the regulations are presented, comprehension eases the way to compliance.

It is important not to underestimate the importance of the planning process. GMP compliance will involve many people from different departments, and various parts of the plan will frequently overlap, both in content and in time interval. Using a Gantt chart (Figure 2.1) optimizes utilization of manpower, budget, and time.

2.3.2 Documenting the progress

Once the plan has been accepted, the budget approved, and the manpower assigned, the project can proceed. Perhaps the most important aspect of any project, and most certainly of a project requiring compliance, is documentation [2]. It is imperative to document all aspects of the project for several reasons: to record all activities, to serve as legal proof (e.g., for a patent), to provide a historical database (for review, trend and yield analysis, etc.) and, finally, to fulfill legal requirements such as the Food, Drug and Cosmetic Act (FD&CA). These reasons are discussed in more detail in Chapter 3, Documentation Systems.

The documentation systems required for GMP production include documentation of the process variables, the specific analytical methods used to determine the quality of the intermediate and final products, and the functioning of the support systems. These support systems include documentation that the facility is suitable and functioning, the specific equipment is clean and functioning, the process is maintained in a reproducible manner, the product is generated without contaminants, and the balance of the quality assurance (QA) systems (i.e., labeling review, records review, nonconforming materials investigation, procedure revision and control, vendor auditing, internal auditing, complaint investigation, etc.) required for GMP compliance are functioning on an on-going basis.

It is usually an accepted concept that the process itself must be documented. Occasionally, however, more naive companies perceive this as a requirement for only postlicensing production, as opposed to being necessary for any clinical production also. These companies may be

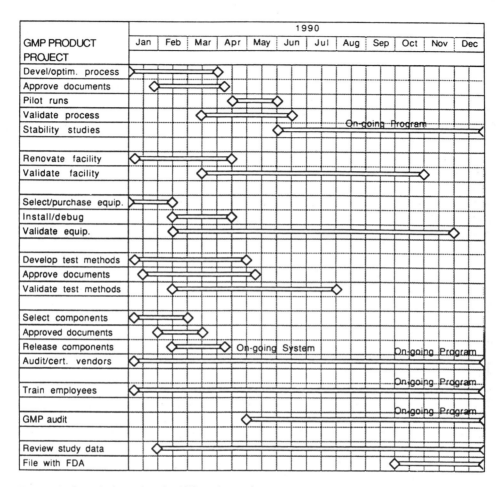

Figure 2.1 Example Gantt chart for GMP product project

tempted to dispense with GMP systems. Common targets for exclusion are: quality control (QC) testing and releasing of raw materials, labeling, and in-process production stages; review of batch records; utilizing double checks; calculating yields; facility and equipment preventative maintenance; equipment calibration; validation; etc.

For some reason, the importance of documentation of analytical methods is not as readily accepted as the requirement to document the production process. Analytical methods of different varieties are used to define and characterize the product. These methods need to be accurate and consistent—they will generate the data that important development decisions are based on. It is important that these decisions, and therefore the methods, be defendable. More details on assay validation can be found in Chapter 7 on statistics, sampling, and analytical method validation.

The validation of facilities and equipment, covered in detail in Chapter 4, and of processes (i.e., reproducibility and contamination minimization) must be documented in a thorough manner. This includes developing operating procedures, calibration procedures, preventive maintenance procedures, and trend charting of monitoring point data. This documentation is critical, even if generating it extends the time necessary to complete the validation. The parameters and conditions in place during the validation determine the operating parameters for subsequent runs and future production. Any later changes or variation, however slight they appear, in the operation of equipment, process, or facilities could affect the final product purity and efficacy. The operating ranges, determined during the validation, can eventually form the basis of process optimization and cost reduction.

The documents (i.e., the forms and lists) developed during the validation process for validation data collection and review can continue to be used after the formal validation period and during the production period. Based on the experience gained during validation and early production, it may be necessary to revise or upgrade the documents and the ranges specified. In addition, sometimes the monitoring points and frequency of sampling used during the validation period can be reduced as experience and confidence in the equipment and system grows. This data, particularly when trend charted, serves as an on-going "revalidation" and also as an "early warning system" of equipment/system failure.

2.3.3   Training for GMP compliance

21 CFR 211.25 lists the requirements for all personnel "engaged in the manufacture, processing, packing, or holding for a drug product" [3]. One of these requirements is training, both in the particular operations that the employee performs and in current GMP.

2.3.3.1   On-the-job training

In addition to fulfilling a GMP requirement, on-the-job training is necessary for consistency of operations and final product. Just as the process, equipment, and facilities are required to be validated to prove that they can function in a consistent and acceptable manner, the personnel also must be "validated" to prove that they are operating the process, equipment, and facilities in a consistent and acceptable manner. The training must be directed by a qualified individual. This individual could be the validation engineer or specialist who performed the validation test runs, the department supervisor who selected, analyzed, and debugged the system, the R&D scientist who developed/validated the process, or even another previously trained and validated employee. In any case, it is important that the qualifications of the trainer be recorded.

In addition to being a technical expert, the trainer should have some background in teaching. It is important to put the specific operations in a broader context to explain the reasons and logic behind the steps, as well as to point out critical aspects. If complex, the operation should be broken down into smaller segments to facilitate learning. It also is important to allow the trainee to perform the operation under the supervision of the trainer. Supportive aspects of the operation (i.e., emergency procedures, local authority for assistance, documentation requirements of the operation, etc.) also need to be included in the training.

As with any validation process, the on-the-job training for each individual must be documented.

2.3.3.2 GMP training

Each employee is required to be trained in the GMP regulations. This training also must be provided by a qualified individual on a continuing basis. The most successful GMP training programs exist in companies where upper management acknowledges the need for a continuing GMP training program. This support includes providing the trainer with a budget for time and materials necessary to establish and maintain an effective and informative GMP training program. There are some films and videotapes commercially available on the subject of GMP. However, to be specific and current, many companies eventually develop a videotape or slides for their own presentations. Even companies without corporate training departments have developed innovative ideas for creative GMP training programs [4]. Some companies use consultants until they have a staff available to provide GMP training.

The last, but perhaps most important, aspect of all types of training is documentation. It is critical that training, as everything else associated with GMP production, be documented. It is helpful if all of the information is available on a database so it is readily available. The database should permit sorting by individual employee, department, function or job operation, type of training, and time period. Data should be available on each course that includes course title/ number, course content or outline, trainer and trainer's qualifications, and date(s) and length of course. Since GMP training is required to be ongoing, the database should be capable of identifying come-up dates to schedule retraining.

Recently, the question of effectiveness of training has been raised. Perhaps the most straightforward determination of effectiveness of training is testing. However, using tests raises other issues: What is the validity of the test? What, if any, subsequent use exists for test results for purposes other than verification of training? The selection of an employee certification method should be reviewed carefully by upper management.

2.3.4 Auditing the progress

In an R&D operation or even a small start-up company, it may be possible for one person to perform or at least supervise all of the aspects necessary for the production and testing of a product. However, as the operation grows, it is no longer likely that a single individual is knowledgeable in all functions or confident of the level of quality employed during all operations. Therefore, systems must be set up for the accumulation of data and for the review of that data. In addition, the systems themselves must be reviewed, or audited, to determine that they are still operating as originally planned.

The Food and Drug Administration (FDA) is aware of the necessity of the review and auditing process. The initial review is usually called the Production Record Review, and is specified in 21 CFR 211.192. This section requires that QA review all records associated with the production of each lot, as well as any discrepancies, and extend that review to other lots possibly involved.

All aspects of the process should be audited. Depending on the size of the operation, it may be necessary to spread the audit over an extended time period. All aspects of production should be audited: raw material receipt and handling, component preparation, fermentation, purification, aseptic materials preparation, final filtration, filling, lyophilization, packaging, shipping, etc. All aspects of QA should be audited: raw material testing, in-process testing and controls, biological assays, biochemical assays, environmental monitoring, trend charting, labeling controls, investigation reports, production records review, annual reviews, stability data, complaint files, etc. All aspects of any support system should be audited: utilities generation and control, computer controls, preventive maintenance, calibration, sanitation, distribution records, etc.

The frequency of internal audits is a subject that should be addressed by the company. An annual audit is probably reasonable for an established operation that shows no major, unexplained product or process failures. A newer operation might be audited more frequently, and a less critical operation less frequently.

2.3.4.1 Audit policy

The "GMPs for Medical Devices" were promulgated after the Section 211 General GMPs. A more extensive audit is required by medical device GMP [5] and by Good Laboratory Practices (GLP) [6] than the initial review of the production records specified in 21 CFR 211.192. As a consequence of the current application of GMP philosophy, the requirement for internal audits has been applied, both by the industry and by the FDA, to all types of pharmaceutical production. The formal audit program must meet the standard expectations of any formal GMP-compliant system: it must be written, it must be organized (i.e., planned and periodic), it must follow approved procedures, and the auditors must be trained and not have direct responsibility for the area being audited. The results of the audit must be reviewed by upper management as delineated in the audit policy. Any corrective actions dictated by the findings of the audit should be completed and a re-audit performed when indicated. All of the auditing activities should be documented.

The medical device GMPs state that an FDA employee shall have access to the operating procedures established for the auditing and that the manufacturer, upon request, shall certify that the program is functioning, documented, and that any required corrective actions have been taken. In lieu of such certification, it may be possible to show the audit log (or history) to demonstrate that the system is in compliance.

An overall site audit will mimic a thorough regulatory agency inspection. An initial review of administrative details, such as the scope/extent and timing of the audit, any restrictions to be conformed to, degree of participation by on-site staff, etc., is recommended to establish a common basis of understanding. An initial review of administrative paperwork, such as organizational charts, list of QA responsibilities, site blueprints, product lists, site/company policies, etc., is an excellent starting point to familiarize the auditor with the current status of the site.

The incoming raw materials handling system should be reviewed. Attention should be given to the physical aspects of material flow, segregation and separation, and reject and returned product holding areas. Other issues to be reviewed are: material status labeling, sampling environment and controls, testing requirements, paperwork flow, and release mechanisms. If automated controls are used, their validation should be reviewed. The warehouse environmental controls, as well as those of any constant temperature holding areas, should be reviewed.

The production process should be reviewed from start to finish, including compliance to Investigational New Drugs (IND), New Drug Applications (NDA), etc.; product and people flow; compliance to Batch Production Records (BPR); process and environmental controls; equipment calibration; preventative maintenance; cleaning; product and equipment status labeling and usage; validation of process, facility and equipment; etc. The QA/QC department should be audited for compliance to established, validated methods; use of approved procedures; documentation practices; review of each lot's manufacturing, testing and release records; review of discrepancies and investigations; annual review of records; stability program; product complaint investigation system; etc.

The distribution system should be reviewed for compliance to standard operating procedures (SOP), for compliance of records, and for availability and compliance of specific systems such as recall, product complaints, and product returns, etc. Any of the support functions not already covered should be addressed: sanitization system and records, employee training program and records, procedure approval and revisions system and historical files, BPR generation system and records, etc.

An overall audit by an internal auditor usually is scheduled for a longer time period than a regulatory agency audit, since the purpose of the internal audit is to anticipate problems (or situations before they become problems) and to assure upper management that all systems are in compliance. Since the internal auditor is usually privy to the site's current status and situations, the auditor can usually probe to the noncompliance issues quickly.

2.3.4.2 Documentation associated with auditing

The first type of documentation associated with auditing is the master schedule. This is usually generated in advance, sometimes up to one or two years for the more complex or structured organizations. Sometimes this schedule is included in the audit policy or SOP, but the audit team can be more flexible (and responsive to current problems or situations) if the schedule is not included in specific detail in the audit policy.

Internal audits are traditionally not surprise audits. The audit team can be more efficient if it prepares in advance for the audit and familiarizes itself with the specific operation and the corresponding documentation as much as possible prior to beginning the physical audit. But, no matter how familiar the team is with the operation, the audit will be more efficient with the participation and cooperation of the immediate management team. Advance scheduling can assist in securing cooperation.

The audit team usually makes notations as detailed as possible to aid in subsequent report writing. They also may obtain copies of various documents, records, or reports for the same purpose.

Many audit teams have wrap-up meetings with the management personnel from the area being audited. The frequency of these meetings will depend on the availability of personnel, timing and major purpose of the audit, etc. It is best if a tentative schedule for wrap-up meetings is agreed upon at the beginning of the audit. At the wrap-up meetings, the audit team usually gives a verbal or intermediate report on its findings and perhaps a summary of the status of the audit. The audit team is usually available to discuss GMP concepts and corporate policies and also to suggest possible corrective actions. Communication is very important during both the audit and the wrap-up meetings to eliminate misunderstandings and minimize duplication of efforts. Whether the intermediate wrap-up meetings are documented is an issue for the individual company's practice and policy.

The final audit report, however, should be formally documented and, to maximize its impact, should be available as soon as possible after the audit is completed. Either this report or a summary should be presented to upper management, either by the audit team or the immediate management, depending again on the individual company's practice and policy. If there is a cooperative effort between the audit team and the immediate management, the audit team can usually recommend specific improvements or suggest specific corrective actions. The audit team also can benefit the immediate management by providing other services (i.e., identifying possible vendors, recommending reading material, providing training service, acting as technical consultants, etc.). In a multisite operation, the audit team can insure that similar operations and documentation are performed in a consistent manner. The audit report, either after its initial presentation or subsequently, should have a corrective action plan developed for each discrepancy listed. This plan also should be presented to upper management for information, review, and approval.

The final type of documentation associated with the audit is the audit log. This log summarizes the activities of the audit: date, facility/area being audited, audit team members, status of audit and report, status of corrective actions, etc.

2.3.4.3 Corrective action plan and follow-up

Almost any audit will uncover discrepancies; some may be major and some minor. In any case, all discrepancies should be addressed with a written plan for corrective action. Initially the corrective action plan should address the specific item cited (i.e., the room where the wall surface was cracked, the SOP that had the inconsistent section, etc.), but, in addition to addressing the specific item, the corrective action should address the cause of the problem and develop a plan to prevent reoccurrence (i.e., establish an annual program for repainting, establish a schedule for routine review of SOPs, etc.).

In addition to establishing corrective action to be taken, the plan should contain an anticipated completion date for each corrective action. The anticipated completion date should be realistic in that it is feasible to achieve and reasonable in that it is timely. If many items are cited in the report, it is unrealistic to expect they all will be completed within a few days. On the other hand, neither is it reasonable to cite a date one to two years in the future just to assure that all actions will be completed well before the date cited.

It is usually the audit team's responsibility to monitor the progress of the corrective action. This follow-up is frequently in the form of a quarterly progress report or phone call. The audit team can be helpful during the period of corrective action. If a corrective action has not been completed, funded, etc., the audit team may be able to suggest an alternative but comparable corrective action or a different approach to complete the original action.

Once corrective actions have been completed, most companies elect to destroy the audit report (and corresponding notes). The audit log, however, should be maintained to aid future scheduling and provide data if certification of compliance to the audit program is required by the FDA.

2.3.4.4 Confidentiality

As mentioned earlier, the GMP regulations do permit the FDA to assure themselves that an audit program is functioning. It is currently the FDA's administrative policy not to request access to the results of the internal audits during routine inspections to determine compliance with current GMP (cGMP) or GLP regulations [7].

2.4 Conclusion

Perhaps the most appropriate definition of GMP is "Doing it right the first time." The GMP regulations can be considered an excellent business outline: they list the steps necessary to produce a product in a consistent fashion, under control, and with acceptable and consistent quality. If each of these steps is followed in a logical fashion, the product will be produced and tested efficiently, and in compliance with the GMP regulations. As stated by Henry Avallone, FDA Mid-Atlantic Region, "...it is important to practice good science in the manufacture and control of clinical products. Manufacturers who are committed to good science and who have a genuine concern about the safety of the person who will be given the investigational drug will have little problem complying with the law."

References

[1]   Chew, N.J. "Regulatory Affairs: Now It's Your Turn." *BioPharm* (Nov./Dec. 1990).

[2]   Vasilevsky, M. and Cherry, C.W. "Documentation Requirements in the Biotechnology Industry." *BioPharm* (Oct. 1990).

[3]   "Personnel Qualifications." Title 21, Code of Federal Regulations, Section 211.25. Washington, DC: Office of the Federal Register, National Archives and Records Administration, 1989.

[4]   Immel, B. "More Creative Ideas for GMP Training." *Medical Device and Diagnostic Industry* (June 1989).

[5]   Immel, B. "GMP Training from the Employees' Perspective." *Medical Device and Diagnostic Industry* (June 1990).

[6]   "Audit Procedures." Title 21, Code of Federal Regulations, Section 820.20(B). Washington, DC: Office of the Federal Register, National Archives and Records Administration, 1989.

[7]   "Quality Assurance Unit." Title 21, Code of Federal Regulations, Section 58.35. Washington, DC: Office of the Federal Register, National Archives and Records Administration, 1989.

[8]   *Federal Register 54*(56), (24 Mar. 1989).

3 Documentation systems

C. Brochard

Contents

3.1   Purpose of documentation

The first protein produced from a recombinantly derived cell was made in 1974. Since that time, there have been fewer than a dozen licensed products developed using this technology. Clearly the experience the biotechnology industry has had in bringing processes into current good manufacturing practice (cGMP) has been quite limited. The challenge of establishing cGMP in this environment is very different from the traditional pharmaceutical company in many ways.

The challenge that biotechnology companies face is to establish the same degree of cGMP compliance as larger pharmaceutical companies. This generally has to be done with somewhat limited resources and staffs largely composed of research and development (R&D) scientists with little or no experience in cGMPs. Documentation is probably the first cGMP requirement that is needed and perhaps the most important.

Documentation serves three fundamental purposes:

1. It can provide good project planning tools which can improve communication of project goals and priorities.
2. It provides an historical record to demonstrate to others what was done, how it was done, what was changed, who did it, when it occurred, and why it was done. Without a good historical perspective, sound decisions on process changes cannot be made.
3. It is required by the cGMP. These regulations clearly recognize that documentation makes good common sense. For those who have experienced cGMP audits, "if it is not documented, it did not happen."

Due to the developmental nature of the biotechnology industry, the need for record keeping is frequently overlooked. As a new product is developed, documentation is often viewed as a burden inhibiting the progress of the project. Unfortunately, this misconception can cause delays in even the earliest stages of development. For example, without some form of documentation, it would not be possible to reproduce methods developed in one laboratory in another. In the extreme case, inadequate documentation may lead to needlessly repeated experiments or to faulty conclusions.

3.2   Types and purposes of documents and documentation

3.2.1   Project scope and management

The earliest form of documentation needed in developing a new product is a description of the scope and goal of the project. This document usually takes the form of a project timeline or Gantt chart. This planning tool is constructed first by breaking down the various stages in the project and listing them in their approximate chronological order. Next, the interrelationships between the various stages are determined to help identify activities which depend on the completion of others. Using the order of events, the chart is constructed by drawing timelines showing the duration of each stage and indicating which stages are dependent on completion of other stages (Figure 3.1 on next page). Another feature of a Gantt chart is to show who is responsible for each stage of the project. The chart can be updated throughout the life of the project to track its progress.

This method of project planning is used almost universally and does an excellent job of highlighting the important stages of the project. From the example in Figure 3.1, the project stage "documentation" spans a large period of time and has important interrelationships with several project milestones.

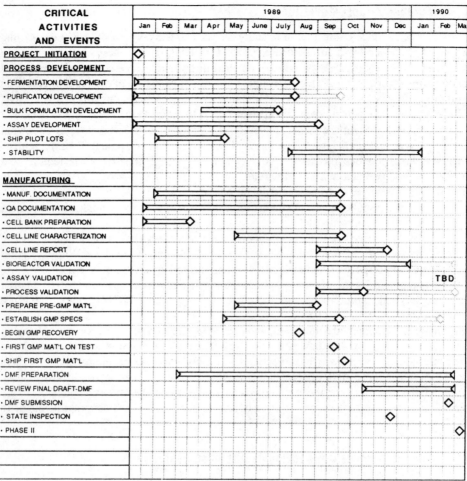

CRITICAL ACTIVITIES AND EVENTS	1989												1990		
	Jan	Feb	Mar	Apr	May	June	July	Aug	Sep	Oct	Nov	Dec	Jan	Feb	Ma
PROJECT INITIATION															
PROCESS DEVELOPMENT															
· FERMENTATION DEVELOPMENT															
· PURIFICATION DEVELOPMENT															
· BULK FORMULATION DEVELOPMENT															
· ASSAY DEVELOPMENT															
· SHIP PILOT LOTS															
· STABILITY															
MANUFACTURING															
· MANUF. DOCUMENTATION															
· QA DOCUMENTATION															
· CELL BANK PREPARATION															
· CELL LINE CHARACTERIZATION															
· CELL LINE REPORT															
· BIOREACTOR VALIDATION															
· ASSAY VALIDATION													TBD		
· PROCESS VALIDATION															
· PREPARE PRE-GMP MAT'L															
· ESTABLISH GMP SPECS															
· BEGIN GMP RECOVERY															
· FIRST GMP MAT'L ON TEST															
· SHIP FIRST GMP MAT'L															
· DMF PREPARATION															
· REVIEW FINAL DRAFT-DMF															
· DMF SUBMISSION															
· STATE INSPECTION															
· PHASE II															

Figure 3.1   Gantt chart showing a project timeline

Thursday, November 15, 1990

3.2.2   Process overview

The first area of documentation described on the Gantt chart is the process overview, which can be developed in a variety of formats that all serve the same function. Process overview is designed to explain the major process steps in sufficient detail so that people who will be involved with document development, regulatory submissions, quality assurance (QA), or engineering may understand how the product will be made so they can anticipate needs and better perform their work. While writing this document, the scientists in process development are creating what will become the "blueprint" of the future process. At this early stage, it is unlikely that the process limits, which are required for clinical product, will be established. What should be included are the process target values required at each step. A good format to use for the process overview can be as follows:

1. PURPOSE: a brief summary of the procedures which will be used to produce the product,
    a. type of cell used for production, and
    b. downstream purification steps.
2. REQUIRED RESOURCES: a description of the raw materials, facilities, major equipment, personnel requirements, and test methods that will be used.
3. PROCESS OUTLINE: a step-by-step description of the process including references to specific materials, equipment, and methods used. Process Flow Charts are an excellent addition to this section.
4. PRODUCT CHARACTERIZATION: a list of tests that are performed to assure the purity, integrity, and strength of the in-process and final container product.
5. CHANGE AUTHORITY: a statement describing the method for controlling process changes and the individuals required to review and approve changes. This will help assure that the product produced at the beginning of process development is equivalent to the final process.

The advantage of developing a good overview is that it sets up the framework for developing documents for several other purposes. It can be used as the basis for filing regulatory documents such as the drug master file (DMF) or the filing of the investigational new drug (IND) document. Similarly, the process overview can help the production standard operating procedures (SOP) and QA testing documents evolve into an integrated system.

3.2.3 Research notebook

The research notebook is the first level of documentation usually found within the biotechnology research environment and should not be overlooked. A well-organized notebook documenting the experiments performed during process development can serve as excellent support for process validation. Details of these experiments can prove useful in determining validation limits and, ultimately, process limits. In fact, process procedures are frequently extracted from research notebooks and used as the basis for what the process will become. With this in mind, the structure and organization of the notebook should be designed to meet those needs.

The research notebook should be bound, with prenumbered pages. It is also a good practice to number the notebook itself and to maintain issuance records to track who received it and for what purpose. The investigator should title the book and include a signature page.

The most important part of the research notebook is the table of contents. A good table of contents will ease retrieval of information by the investigator, as well as others, long after the experiments are completed. It should include the date work was performed, project identification, what was performed, and the page numbers used.

It is also a good practice to include a preface for the notebook to help define its scope and purpose. Information that might be included is the goal of the work, who will perform the work, where the work will be performed, where the analysis will be performed, where any supporting information may be located, and how it can be identified.

The text within the notebook can take many forms, but a preferred format consists of the following five elements:

1. INTRODUCTION: statement of purpose and brief explanation of what will be done.
2. EXPERIMENTAL PLAN: gives a forward look of what is planned to be done and what methods and instruments will be used. It is also a good idea to include contingency plans to link subsequent experiments.

3. OBSERVATIONS AND DATA: record of raw data collection and experimental observations which can help others repeat what was done.
4. DISCUSSION OF RESULTS: perform data reduction and develop supporting information for conclusions.
5. CONCLUSION: state whether or not the experimental goals were reached, the strength of the results, and if any future experiments are planned.

3.2.4 SOPs

Once the process has become stabilized and the experimentation begins to diminish, it is appropriate to begin defining the process using SOPs. These procedures should be designed to assure reproducibility of the process and, hence, the quality and integrity of the material produced. They should be written with sufficient detail to permit individuals practiced in the techniques to reproducibly manufacture the product. However, they should not be so restrictive as to limit small changes but must emphasize areas where a change could affect the quality of the product. The SOP can be thought of as a "bridging document" that standardizes the techniques used in the process development and begins defining the process to be used for clinical manufacture or production. These documents differ from laboratory notebooks because they are prewritten, standardized, and contain detailed instruction. They differ from documents that would be used for clinical production because data is usually recorded in research notebooks along with any process deviations or observations. Frequently at this stage of development, more process and testing information is gathered than is normally required in a production document. The flexibility provided by the research notebook is needed to record this information.

There are many valuable things to be learned during the preparation of SOPs. While writing them, people are forced to think through the process and may frequently discover or anticipate problems that otherwise might have caused costly problems after scale-up of the process. Once written, SOPs will help standardize the training of technicians who will be running the process and minimize any misunderstanding of how things are to be done. Once the standard methods are established, it is possible to evaluate empirically if process improvements or changes can be made without affecting the quality or integrity of the product. If process changes are made, the SOP's history file (which will be discussed later) serves as tracking mechanism for changes. Each new SOP becomes a training tool and a communication device for those using them. Another important function of the SOP is to tell the user what needs to be recorded.

Without careful documentation of the operation, well-conceived processes will be of limited value. Just as a carefully run laboratory experiment is documented in a notebook, so must the process information be recorded. In Section 3.2.5, examples of how and what kind of information should be recorded are given. SOP documents are typically used during the preclinical production phase and then further refined into batch production records (BPRs), which are used for clinical production under the cGMP regulations.

3.2.5 Documentation for testing

Following a parallel path, the documents describing the test procedures found within the analytical development laboratory and QA laboratory also take on a more formal approach. Written SOPs in the laboratory standardize the test methods by identifying the methods, standards, equipment, and reagents used. This standardization, as in the production process, assures that each time the test is performed, results will be consistent, and the variation from operator to operator will be minimized. Laboratory test methods also should include the use of positive and negative controls to confirm the validity of assay results. The testing SOP should outline the data and test values that should be recorded in the notebook. Specific test values can be recorded to permit process monitoring and evaluation of assay performance.

As the process evolves further toward production of clinical product, the documentation requirements become more stringent. The cGMPs outline the requirements for records and record keeping in the 21 CFR 211.180 through 211.194. In these subsections, the requirements for documentation are more directed toward the production and control of a series of batches of product. Records are used for more than documenting the current lot or test. If properly set up, the document system can be used for trend analysis and process review. In fact, this purpose is specifically described in the cGMPs in subsection 211.180 [3].

3.2.6   BPRs

BPRs are designed to standardize the process like an SOP but also provide lot-specific information. This is typically accomplished by taking the SOPs for each critical step in the process and developing lot-specific record forms to record the information. The following outlines the documentation requirements listed in the 21 CFR 211.180ff:

MASTER PRODUCTION AND CONTROL RECORD (See 211.186)
    a. A record of the production process used including batch size, with double checks at each critical step should be kept.
    b. Include within the production document:
        1. The name and strength of the product,
        2. Identification and reconciliation of the name and weight of each active ingredient used,
        3. A list of all components used with their specific identity,
        4. The quantity of each ingredient added,
        5. A statement if any excess quantity is added,
        6. Calculations showing the actual versus the theoretical measurements and yields,
        7. A description of the container/closure used with an actual label specimen, and
        8. Complete instructions for sampling, testing, and storing the product at each stage of the process.

BATCH PRODUCTION AND CONTROL RECORDS (see 21 CFR 211.188)
    Records prepared for each batch should include:
    a. A signed review of the Master Production and Control Records, and
    b. Documentation at each significant step of the following:
        1. Date of the process,
        2. Equipment identity,
        3. The components and in-process materials used,
        4. Quantity of each material used,
        5. In-process and laboratory control results,
        6. Inspection of packaging and label areas before use,
        7. Comparison of actual and theoretical yields,

8. Sample label instructions and label control records,
9. Type of container/closure used,
10. Sampling instructions,
11. Identity of persons performing and supervising each significant step,
12. Investigations and the results of any process excursions, and
13. Inspection of the final product.

This outline summarizes the key points covered in the 21 CFR 211 concerning BPRs. It is recommended that the specific regulations are frequently reviewed during the preparation of procedures. Some details have been omitted here for clarity.

3.3   Good laboratory practice (GLP) documentation

3.3.1   Planning for preclinical documents

From the preceding outline of the documentation required for clinical grade product, it is apparent that several types of documents need to be set up during the preclinical operations. A document system should be organized to permit efficient use by the various groups involved. An index with a logical document numbering system is helpful in retrieving documents and maintaining the system. The index and numbering system should separate the documents by:

1. Functional group (e.g., testing versus processing),
2. Stage of the process (e.g., fermentation versus purification), and
3. Type (e.g., general procedures versus specific) or product type.

The document numbering system should be flexible enough to accommodate many types of documents. It should also permit the insertion of new or deletion of old documents without disrupting the whole system. It also is extremely important to include in the index the effective date and the revision number of the document to help keep the procedure manuals current.

Just as important as creating an integrated document system is the need to set up a batch or lot number system. A system should be designed to cover every aspect of the process: raw materials, in-process media and reagents, product in process, or standards prepared in QA. The lot numbers should be concise to minimize writing but also should permit easy identification. For example, sometimes it is helpful to build in a date code or a product code to help identify when or what kind of sample was taken. The batch and lot numbers also are very important in organizing and filing the documents required for assembling the lot packet, which will be discussed later.

A formal system of review, approval, and revision also should be set up to control the issuance of the documents. At a minimum, each one should be reviewed by a technical person involved with process development, a production person, and a QA person. The review should be documented on a record (Figure 3.2) with the signature of the persons responsible and any comments made. This record also should include the reason the document is needed or why revision is necessary. The combination of this record and all revisions of the document should be filed together to create the history file.

Document appearance is a frequently overlooked detail that has a large impact on long-term acceptance. A consensus should be reached by all of the users for the most acceptable format. This is especially true for the BPRs. Some people prefer to have documents that integrate the data with the text; others prefer to keep text and data separate. In the first case, keeping the text and record form together insures that the technician performing the work has the current procedure

Document No _____
Revision No._____to_____

Request for document change

Document type: [ ] QA   [ ] Production   [ ] Other

Document status: [ ] New   [ ] Revised   [ ] Killed

Date needed:_____

Describe document or reason for change (attach additional pages if required):

Requester:_____Date: _____

Route to next person after review.
        Name   Date   Response

1)_____   _____   1   2   3

2)_____   _____   1   2   3

3)_____   _____   1   2   3

4)_____   _____   1   2   3

Please review the attached document, sign and indicate your response or comments if any.

Responses: 1) Accept document as is.
                2) Suggest the following changes but acceptable as is.
                3) Unacceptable unless the following changes are made.

Comments:

Figure 3.2 Documentation review record

present at all times. The drawback is that the BPRs can be rather lengthy, and retrieval of process data becomes difficult. Fortunately, compromises are possible to take advantage of either format. Document appearance is somewhat computer and software dependent. It is a good idea to plan ahead and install the equipment needed in the long-term so a consistent format can be maintained (Figure 3.3).

SOP No. XX-XXX
Revision No. Draft   Lot # _____

**Title: Preparation of Sterile   Date Effective:_____
           Aliquots of 1X Trypsin-EDTA
                                            Prepared by:_____
Approved by:
Production_____   Quality Assurance_____**

---

1.   Prepare work area per Procedure No. XX-XXX: Preparing Tissue Culture Work Area.

Work area prepared by: _____   Date: _____

2.   Thaw a tube of 10X Trypsin-EDTA (5mL). Aseptically add 45 mL of PBS (Ca^{2+} and Mg^{2+} free) to
        the 10X Trypsin.

10X Trypsin-EDTA (BPR XX-XXX) Lot # _____

PBS   Raw Material ID#_____ Vol: _____mL added by: _____

3.   Filter-sterilize 1X Trypsin using a 0.2 μm filter unit and store in a sterile 50 mL tube.

Filter Used: Raw Material ID#_____   By: _____ .

4.   Label tube as follows: (Attach sample label)

        1X Trypsin-EDTA   Lot #
        Date Filter Sterilized
        Expiration Date   (Note: Expiration is four weeks from date of filter sterilization.)
        Operator

                                            Labeled by: _____ Date_____

5.   Store at 2-8°C.

                                            Stored by: _____ Date_____

Note: 1X Trypsin-EDTA may be used up to 4 weeks when stored at 2-8 °C. Check solution for turbidity
and discard if cloudy.

6.   Record use of 1X Trypsin-EDTA on Material Accountability Sheet or tracking card.

REVIEW RECORD	
All Pages Present . . . . ( )	Current Revision Used. . . . . ( )
Batch # in Red on Each Page . . .( )	Duplicating Quality Acceptable . . . . ( )
Reviewed By: _____Date: _____	Audited By: _____ Date: _____

Comments: _____
_____

Figure 3.3 Example of computer-formatted BPR

3.3.2 Getting started

3.3.2.1 Raw material documents

After the decisions are made for setting up the document system, one of the first activities should
be cataloguing raw materials. From the process overview created in process development, make

a list of all the required raw materials. From this list, unique raw material identity numbers can be assigned for each material for processing and document purposes. The first set of documents should establish the specifications and acceptance criteria for the raw materials. During the preclinical phase, the testing requirements for these materials will be established and laboratory procedures developed.

Typically, materials are tested visually, chemically, and microbiologically to insure their identity and purity before use. Methods are usually adapted from standard compendial methods such as the United States Pharmacopeia (USP) and the American Chemical Society (ACS). In the early phases, these materials are frequently tested by outside test facilities before methods are developed in-house. This does not relieve the manufacturer of the requirement of establishing specifications, methods, and procedures for evaluating the materials.

3.3.2.2 Sampling documents
The next area that requires early attention is selection of the steps in the process where sampling and testing will be required. Sampling plans should be set up that will assure the process is monitored so that the purity, integrity, stability, and yields of the product are documented. Examples of the kinds of testing performed might include microbiological and endotoxin testing of the culture media, enzyme-linked immunosorbent assay (ELISA) activity in the harvest, polyacrylamide gel electrophoresis (PAGE) and high-pressure liquid chromatography (HPLC) performed during and after purification, peptide maps, and n-terminal sequences to confirm identity.

These plans should contain sufficient information so that the person sampling knows exactly how much to sample, what kind of container to use, how it should be labeled, how it should be stored, and what kind of testing should be performed. Similar to raw materials, laboratory test methods must be documented and the methods validated to show that they have an acceptable degree of accuracy and precision to assure that the process is in control.

3.3.2.3 Laboratory documents
Almost simultaneous to the development of sampling plans, laboratory documents must be developed for the raw materials and in-process testing. As mentioned previously, it is good practice to use the accepted methodology outlined in the USP and the ACS. These methods lend themselves very well to the formats described here.

In addition, laboratory documents also should meet the requirements outlined in 21 CFR 211.194. The important features are summarized below:

1. Record forms should include a description of the sample, identifying where it was taken, how much was sampled, who sampled it, the lot number, date sampled, date received, date tested, and method used.
2. Test procedures must include some estimation of precision and accuracy if the method is not a compendial method. If the method is adapted from a compendial method, some evidence of suitability for the specific use must be included. A validation protocol and acceptance report should be issued for each noncompendial analytical method. (Note: It is generally expected that each assay's precision and accuracy have been determined or validated and that positive and negative controls are included to assure the validity of each assay. See Chapter 7 for further discussion.)
3. Location of all original test data must be identified on the test record. Traceability to any reagents used must be included.

4. Copies of any calculations used to arrive at the test result must be included in the record. Test results, acceptance criteria, and a review by a responsible individual also should be included.
5. Laboratory records should be developed for the preparation, standardization, and use of any laboratory standards. For example, logbooks should be maintained documenting the receipt and release of chemicals used in testing and recording how reagent solutions are prepared.
6. Calibration records are required for lab instruments, test apparatus, gauges, and recording devices.
7. Documentation of training for laboratory personnel is required to assure that testing is performed by individuals who are technically competent and knowledgeable in the GMPs.

These items comprise the minimum documentation requirement required for test records. It is quite apparent from this list that the needs for documentation have evolved from simple notebook entries at the R&D or process development stage to a specific list of requirements at the clinical production stage. Figures 3.4 and 3.5 are examples of a simple laboratory procedure and test record.

3.3.2.4 Documents for special circumstances
The goal of performing in-process testing is to assure that the final product meets all desired quality characteristics. This can be accomplished by gathering sufficient test data at strategic points in the process and establishing process control limits. If the process consistently meets these limits, then the final product will be assured of meeting the final product specifications. Because of this need for control of in process variables, it is extremely important that process deviations are handled properly and documented very well. Procedures are needed to explain how to disposition materials that do not conform to in-process limits and assure appropriate corrective action to prevent recurrence.

The procedure should describe who should review the data, what things should be considered in the review, and who should disposition the product. It also should offer specific guidelines to determine if the product produced is equivalent to what was acceptable previously. Some things to consider are:

1. Was the limit properly set?
2. Was the testing performed correctly?
3. Was the process properly validated?
4. Will acceptance of the material impact any of the steps downstream?
5. Are the process documents at fault? Do they need revision?
6. Is additional training required by the technicians performing the process?
7. Is this an isolated incident or are there other lots involved?
8. Is the corrective action likely to prevent recurrence?

These questions must be covered in this procedure. The answers should be included in a report and compiled with the information included with the lot history file.

Another inevitable occurrence with a developing process is change. Despite the fact that the process has become more standardized, changes will naturally occur because of alterations in scale, process improvements, expanded or narrower limits, changes in raw materials, or many other causes. Specific guidelines must be in place to help establish consistent criteria to evaluate each change and its effect. The individuals responsible for reviewing changes must consider the

---

Doc. No. **QA XX-XXX**   Revision No. Draft

Title: **Protein Determination by**   Date Effective:_____
      the Ninhydrin Reaction

                                Prepared by:_____

Approved by:
QA Director _____   **QA Manager** _____

1. Purpose:

    1.1   To determine the presence of protein in solution.

2. References:

    2.1   USP XXII

3. Definitions and Abbreviations:

    3.1   Purified water -- water which meets or exceeds the requirements for Purified Water defined in the USP.

4. Materials:

    4.1   Purified water
    4.2   Triketohydrindene Hydrate TS

5. Equipment:

    5.1   Clean glassware for solution preparation
    5.2   Filter paper, qualitative #1 or equivalent
    5.3   Drying oven, vacuum or equivalent

6. Procedures:

    6.1   Label any stock solutions prepared with the following:

        Solution composition
        Formulator's initials
        Date formulated
        Expiration date

    6.2   Record solutions prepared in the Laboratory Solutions Notebook.

    6.3   Preparation of Stock, Standard and Test Solutions:

        6.3.1   Prepare fresh, Ninhydrin TS by dissolving 200 mg of triketohydrindene hydrate in purified water to make 10 mL.

    6.4   Procedure:

        6.4.1   Reaction with Ninhydrin:
        a)   Place 1 mL of the test solution onto the filter paper and then add 1 mL of the Ninhydrin TS to the same spot on the filter paper.
        b)   Dry in a drying oven at about 105°C for 10 minutes.

7. Interpretation and disposition of results:

    7.1   To positively identify the presence of protein, the residue should turn blue. Report the results as positive or negative for the presence of protein on test record XX-XXX

Figure 3.4 Documentation of a simple laboratory procedure

impact the change will have and set up some method of identifying when it took effect and what lots are involved. A formal system must be established to log these changes, regardless of how insignificant they may appear, to permit any retrospective analysis that may become necessary. Once the process has undergone a thorough characterization or validation, the SOPs are in place, and product specifications are established, it is appropriate to prepare the cGMP documents. In some cases, parts of these studies may be done concurrently with phase I clinical studies.

Document No. QA XX-XXX
Revision No. DRAFT

**Detection of Protein
by
Ninhyrdrin Reaction**

Test Summary Sheet:

Material Tested:_____

Preparation of reagents:

    Materials used: Triketohydrindene hydrate, TS
                Manufactured by:_____Lot#:_____

                Type of filter paper:_____

    Quantity of 0.2% Ninhydrin Solution Prepared:_____

                Outdate:_____

Interpretation and disposition of results:

    Presence of protein in the sample is confirmed if the residue turns blue. Indicate by
    circling the results below.

        Protein   No Protein
        Detected   Detected

Performed By: _____   Date: _____

Reviewed By: _____   Date: _____

Figure 3.5   Documentation of laboratory test summary record

3.4   GMP documentation

3.4.1   Completing what was started

The records required for cGMP are generally an extension of what was started for preclinical production. Following the guidelines outlined in the CFR, the BPRs used for cGMP are designed to simplify the record keeping requirements by including prompts where information is required. During the preclinical production, more reliance is placed on the research notebook where methods and observations are frequently recorded by hand. Since the process has become more standardized and predictable, it is possible to outline the procedure and the expected outcome for each process step and minimize the need to record observations. Nevertheless, a comment section is still a good idea since the unexpected can still happen and observations of the technicians are valuable aids to troubleshooting when necessary.

Another difference between the research notebook and the BPR is the more formal and standardized use of raw materials. The use of QA-tested raw materials is a cGMP requirement. BPRs should list the specific raw material catalog number and require an entry for the raw material identity number. This unique number is assigned by QA to indicate that the material has passed all required testing. Recording the expiration date of materials is done to help protect against the use of outdated materials. The raw material identity number also is used to provide traceability and accountability of the materials used. Traceability is provided by the QA-assigned identity number, which refers to the testing performed to release it. Accountability is accomplished by using log sheets for each raw material lot and indicating how much was used and where it was used. The use of a sequential raw material identity number also can provide a system for rotating stock to facilitate the practice of first in/first out.

3.4.2 Review of cGMP documents

As mentioned above, BPRs include prompts for required information such as double checks at critical process steps. These steps include calculation and addition of active ingredients and verification of dilution calculations, yield calculations, or other important measures. The purpose of double checks is to minimize errors at critical steps in the process. Too many double checks, however, can dilute their effectiveness. They should be used judiciously or replaced where possible by direct recording devices.

cGMP documents should include process limits that will help maintain the process under control. If the limits are derived properly, products produced within them should have a high degree of assurance that all final product specifications and performance will be met. Given this fact, it is extremely important that the process is properly characterized or validated to support the limits included in the BPRs. The limits should be stated at the same place in the document where the information is recorded. Some examples of limits include process parameters, such as pH, temperature, volumes, and concentrations. Other limits require input from testing performed in QA testing labs, such as protein concentration and activity for calculation of yields or specific activity, purity of fractions for monitoring column performance, and microbial load and endotoxin levels for monitoring the effectiveness of a cleaning operation. Because of the separation in time between when an operation is performed and when test results are available, it is often difficult to synchronize testing with the production process. Many solutions have been developed to improve communication, including reporting results through electronic mail or performing the testing within production to assure prompt reporting. Regardless of how the information is generated, it is important that the document clearly states which results are needed before proceeding, what are the limits, that the results are double-checked, and the procedure to follow if the test results are out of limits.

After an operation is complete, a series of reviews are required under the cGMPs. The technician responsible for each process step must verify and sign that it was completed, preferably at the time of operation. Next, the line supervisor responsible for the process should review and sign the process documents. Finally, an independent review is performed by QA that includes all process documents, QA documents, and any other supporting documents. With this review scheme, each document is reviewed three times. To insure that these reviews are properly done, a review document should be prepared.

The purpose of the review document is to outline what documents and data are needed to compile what will become the "lot packet". This packet, once assembled, will permit a reviewer to retrieve any information pertaining to a specific lot. A well-conceived review document will link all required process and test documents together with a summary review document. This summary should include a specific list of all BPRs needed for the process, all in-process assays performed, product specifications, and the lot test results.

In addition, a review must be performed on the non-lot-specific data collected to support the process in general. This would include environmental monitoring of the process areas, testing of the water for injection (WFI) system, autoclave charts, incubator and cold room charts, and clean room air balance measurements. This review usually is performed weekly, and the results are correlated with the product produced during the same period. If the results are unfavorable, any product affected would have to be considered nonconforming and carefully evaluated.

After the completion of the document review, the lot packet and associated documents should be filed and protected against loss due to fire, water, or other peril. These documents are extremely valuable from both a legal and a scientific point of view. They are the primary evidence showing that the process was run according to procedure. Because of this fact, the cGMPs require that all lot packets are maintained not less than one year past the date of expiration for a marketed product or three years past the date of last distribution for products without expiration dates (21 CFR 211.180). These records can be kept as originals, copies, microfiche, or other accurate reproductions of the original and must be available for inspection by the Food and Drug Administration (FDA). Different retention requirements are needed for nonclinical records used in support of an application for research and marketing permit, and these are outlined in the 21 CFR 58.195. Records should be maintained no less than two years after the permit is issued. It should be emphasized that these are the minimum requirements. Individual companies must evaluate the risk versus benefit of retaining records longer.

3.4.3 Miscellaneous cGMP records

A few more records are needed to complete the document system required for cGMP. These records are directed toward preventive maintenance, calibration, and usage of equipment used in production. The purpose of documenting the condition and operation of equipment is an extension of the concept of validation. To produce a consistent product, one must show that the equipment used to produce it functions in the same manner as when it was validated. Preventive maintenance records appear very similar to the owner's manual found in each new car. Based on the equipment manufacturer's recommendations, a maintenance schedule is established based on some measure of use such as number of cycles, hours of operation, or changes in performance. The maintenance procedures should outline what needs to be done in general terms and can make liberal use of any available instruction manuals that come with the machine. Any regularly scheduled or emergency maintenance should be documented on an equipment logsheet. It should indicate what was done, when it was done, who performed the work, and what kind of parts were changed.

An activity associated with preventive maintenance is calibration. In many cases, the calibration procedure is included within the maintenance documents or within laboratory procedures. The most important feature to include within the preventive maintenance and calibration documents is the scheduling feature. It is often difficult to keep track of and schedule all of the required activities. Fortunately, several computer software packages are available to simplify this activity.

3.5 Conclusion

The documentation requirements for an emerging product produced by a biotechnology company are defined by the regulations described within the cGMPs. Since biotechnology companies are usually small and directed toward R&D, a lot of effort is required to establish the documentation systems needed to produce a clinical product. A balance needs to be struck between what documentation is desired and what is required at each stage of development. Too much documentation too soon can become very burdensome and can actually inhibit development—too little can create a weak foundation for what will be required later.

One of the fundamental purposes of documentation is to create an historical record of all of the important processing parameters and the associated testing. Without this record, informed decisions cannot be made about evaluating changes made to the process. Through careful review of well-conceived records, it is possible to reconstruct very accurately what took place during the process. This will help predict what the effect of a process change will be. The advantage of having this information available far outweighs the extra effort required to establish the documentation system initially.

Despite the fact that records are required by the cGMPs, the benefits of good documentation can be appreciated through all phases of development of a product through biotechnology. The earlier the concepts of good record keeping can be applied, the easier it will be to implement the required records for cGMP.

References

[1]   Willig, S.H.; Tuckerman, M.M.; and Hitchings, W.S. *Good Manufacturing Practices for Pharmaceuticals.* New York: Marcel Dekker, 1982.

[2]   Title 21, Code of Federal Regulations, Sections 1–99 and 200–299. Washington, DC: Office of the Federal Register, National Archives and Records Administration, 1989.

[3]   Garner, W.Y. and Barge, M.S. *Good Laboratory Practices.* Washington, DC: American Chemical Society, 1988.

[4]   Kanare, H.M. *Writing the Laboratory Notebook.* Washington, DC: American Chemical Society, 1985.

[5]   Bryant, R. *The Pharmaceutical Quality Control Handbook.* Eugene, OR: Aster, 1984.

4 Validation

D. R. Colton

Contents

4.1 Overview of validation

Validation is an essential element of biopharmaceutical manufacturing that begins with the establishment of product specifications. It is through validation that we demonstrate and document that a manufacturing process is under control and capable of consistently producing a product that meets its predetermined specifications.

4.1.1 Philosophy of validation

Webster's defines "valid" as having a conclusion correctly derived from premises and lists several synonyms for the word: sound, cogent, and telling. Synonyms of "validate" include to verify, substantiate, and confirm. The basic philosophy of validation follows directly from its definition. Validation is the tool with which we provide documented evidence that the facilities we build, the equipment we operate, and the standard operating procedures (SOPs) and manufacturing formulae we follow will consistently produce products that meet their predetermined specifications and quality attributes.

The underlying justification for performing validation is that "quality cannot be tested into a product". Rather, quality is the end product of a thoroughly understood, properly designed, implemented, and controlled manufacturing process. And, like the manufacturing process itself, a validation program that is not properly designed, implemented, and controlled will be difficult to manage and may not produce the desired level of product quality assurance (QA).

Validation is a corporate responsibility, and, as such, it is of little significance which department oversees the validation effort. There may in fact be separate groups to validate different parts of the manufacturing process, production equipment, etc. The task of validation may be divided up among process development, engineering, technical services, quality control (QC), and validation groups as appropriate, or it may be handled by a single group, depending on the size of the corporation, number of systems involved, and the breadth of its product lines. Ultimately, the validation test plan or protocol must be reviewed and approved prior to initiating testing by all departments that will be participating in the validation effort, including any support groups that may be required to provide technical assistance.

In the planning phase prior to validation, each department on the validation team should be consulted for input toward defining the scope of the project and test requirements and to commit their resources to the project. During the review and approval process for validation documents, each department representative should assure that the technical content is accurate and that upon completion of the proposed testing, corporate quality, manufacturing, and regulatory requirements will be met. During review of the final validation acceptance report following testing, each department representative should verify that the document is accurate and complete and that the objectives of the validation protocol were indeed met.

4.1.2 Definitions

The following definitions relate to the validation of biochemical and pharmaceutical procedures:

CALIBRATION: Demonstrating that a measuring device produces results within specified limits, in direct comparison to a reference standard device, over an appropriate range of measurements.

CELL SEED: A quantity of cells derived from a single tissue, typically stored in aliquots at -70 °C or below.

CERTIFICATION: An administrative function in which the review and approval process is accomplished as a final step in the validation program.

CONCURRENT VALIDATION: Establishing documented evidence that a process does what it purports to do based upon data gathered during actual implementation of the process.

DRUG PRODUCT: A finished dosage form (e.g., tablet, capsule, solution, small volume parenteral (SVP), etc.) that contains the active ingredient(s). Drug products for the most part are the result of the formulation of materials of established high quality and are subject to published, finalized government regulations.

HVAC: Heating, ventilation, and air conditioning system.

INTERMEDIATE: Any substance, whether isolated or not, that is produced by chemical, physical, or biological action at some stage in the production of the bulk drug substance and that is subsequently used at another stage in the production of that bulk.

INSTALLATION QUALIFICATION (IQ): Documenting that a system has been installed in adherence with all key design specifications.

MASTER WORKING CELL BANK (MWCB): A quantity of cells of uniform composition, derived from one or more ampoules of the cell seed, stored at -70 °C or below.

OPERATIONAL QUALIFICATION (OQ): Documenting that a system performs as designed throughout all anticipated operating ranges.

PERFORMANCE QUALIFICATION (PQ): An approved plan that will be performed to validate a system or process.

POPULATION DOUBLING LEVEL (PDL): The number of population doublings that a cell culture has undergone.

PROCESS VALIDATION: Establishing documented evidence which provides a high degree of assurance that a specific process will consistently produce a product meeting its predetermined specifications and quality attributes [1].

PROSPECTIVE VALIDATION: Establishing documented evidence prior to process implementation that a process does what it purports to do.

QUALIFICATION: A part of the validation program whereby the physical parametric control of a manufacturing system is evaluated to demonstrate its suitability to carry out the designed process, as separate from validation of the process itself (see IQ and OQ).

4.1.3 Regulatory requirements

The U.S. Food and Drug Administration (FDA) is the governmental regulatory agency that has among its charter the responsibility to assure the safety and efficacy of the drug supply for the American public. The FDA draws its legal authority from the text of Section 501(a)(2)(B) of the Federal Food, Drug, and Cosmetic Act (FD&CA), the good manufacturing practices (GMPs), approved in 1962 [2]. The drug manufacturer is bound to adhere to the GMPs to assure that a drug "meets the requirements of the act as to safety, and has the identity and strength and meets the quality and purity characteristics that is purports or is represented to possess" [3].

Parts 210 and 211 of the GMPs contain the definitions and guidelines by which the FDA may deem that a drug is adulterated and, therefore, take actions against the drug's manufacturer. The actual requirement for process validation comes from the text of Section 211.100 where it is stated that "there shall be written procedures for production and process control designed to assure that the drug products have the identity, strength, quality, and purity they purport or are represented to possess" [4].

In the experience of the author, over the past several years the FDA has gone to great lengths to train its inspectors in the production technologies unique to biopharmaceutical production. Corporations have opened their doors to the FDA to both educate the inspectors and to gain insights into what the FDA's requirements would be for licensing of biopharmaceutical production facilities. One of the developments of this mutual training venture and of the many inspection findings of FDA investigators was the draft "Biotech Inspection Outline" [5]. The outline provides the FDA investigators with questions that are specifically targeted at biopharmaceutical production. This outline and other reference documents regarding government regulations toward drug production are readily available to any manufacturer who needs them. These reference materials should be studied and applied to the individual manufacturer's specific products and production technologies.

4.1.4 Process development

Process development prior to validation testing is crucial to the success of a validation project. Weak or inadequate process development will become obvious through failed validation testing and inconsistent results from manufacturing runs. Planning, foresight, and follow through are what is required to assure that a process is ready for validation and, likewise, implementation into manufacturing use. Validation, QC, QA, process development, manufacturing, and engineering staff must be jointly involved up front to assure the successful development, validation, and ultimate implementation of a process into routine manufacturing.

4.1.5 Change control and revalidation

Change control and revalidation go hand-in-hand. The purpose of having a change control policy is to insure that the integrity of the validated status of systems and procedures is maintained. When changes are required or new procedures are to be implemented, the change control program will be used to evaluate the need for and scope of revalidation testing. Instances requiring revalidation include changes to the production system, product formulation, manufacturing process, equipment, control software, packaging, and the manufacturing facility.

The various departments that have been involved with validation up to this point should have procedures (SOPs) in place to maintain the validated status of manufacturing methods and equipment. These procedures should include periodic audits, routine training of personnel, QC testing, preventive maintenance of equipment, periodic calibration of critical process instrumentation, and periodic review of SOPs. These procedures are essential in a long-term commitment to maintain validation status and process control.

The potential effect of a change to a manufacturing step, be it process or engineering, should be evaluated and a written revalidation plan drafted, if necessary. Revalidation testing should encompass all affected areas of system performance and documentation, including any new information that comes about due to the change. Engineering drawings and manufacturing and preventive maintenance SOPs should be reviewed and amended as required by the change. All document amendments should be approved by the appropriate individuals. Prior validation and manufacturing histories should be consulted for system specifications and operational performance prior to making the change. It may be useful to apply some of this information toward evaluating the effect of the change and the need for revalidation.

4.2   General system and process validation

Production facility design, process equipment design, environmental control, cleaning, and sterilization procedures help assure consistency in the manufacturing process and provide protection of the product from contaminants during processing. Such contaminants may consist of, but are not limited to, virus, endotoxin, bacteria, mycoplasma, and foreign materials including equipment cleaning agents and product and cell line cross contamination. Any process, system, or equipment that may affect product quality should be validated.

New systems and equipment should be verified to be correctly installed in accordance with all key design specifications and local codes and to be fully functional throughout all anticipated ranges of operation. These verifications comprise the IQ and OQ. Well-written and thorough purchase specifications will greatly ease the validation effort and assure that the systems and equipment as installed meet the manufacturer's requirements.

4.2.1   Validation of utilities

Validation of utility systems is performed to document that the systems have been installed properly, meeting process design requirements, manufacturer's recommendations, and all applicable codes. The product of the utility should be measured to provide assurance that it meets both the utility specifications and the process requirements. Compressed air should be tested for moisture and airborne microbial, particulate, and hydrocarbon levels. Nitrogen, oxygen, and other gases must be subjected to compendial testing for purity, at a minimum. A sample of condensed pure steam should be tested for conformance to USP water for injection (WFI) chemical and biological specifications [6]. Samples from WFI and purified water systems should be assayed for conformance to USP chemical and biological specifications.

When sampling utilities such as water, steam, and compressed gasses, the samples should be taken from the inlet and outlet of the main processing unit as well as from multiple ports on the distribution system. Utilities should be challenged by testing under conditions of maximum demand where possible to assure that outputs are adequate for the facility systems serviced by these utilities.

4.2.2   Environmental control

The primary purpose of environmental control validation is to provide assurance that facility design and environmental control procedures are sufficient to maintain the environment within defined limits. Environmental requirements will differ from one area to another depending upon the nature of the manufacturing process being performed in the area. The environmental specifications for a buffer preparation area will be different than those for an aseptic processing area. The environmental control requirements for each of these areas, therefore, will be reflected in the facility design and control systems.

Microbial monitoring of surfaces and air quality should be routinely performed. The desired level of environmental control with respect to temperature, humidity, and airborne microbial and particulate quality must be defined and appropriate for the operations conducted in a given area. QC sampling for these environmental control parameters, therefore, should coincide with facility start-up and be maintained throughout the operational life of the facility.

Environmental control is more than just control over physical environmental attributes; it also includes an effective facility sanitizing program. Properly chosen sanitizing agents are an essential part of a comprehensive environmental control program. The two most important considerations in the selection of sanitizing agents are their compatibility with the surfaces and equipment on which they will be used on and their ability to reduce the bioburden on the surfaces to which they are applied.

To establish the effectiveness of a sanitizing agent, the specific microorganisms typical to the manufacturing environment must be known. Validation and routine QC monitoring of the controlled manufacturing environment and work surfaces will provide a detailed knowledge of the type and level of microorganisms commonly found in the particular areas being sanitized. In this way, the acceptability of specific sanitizing agents can be shown. The effectiveness of a sanitizing agent also may be accomplished in the laboratory.

A comprehensive sanitization program includes rotation of the sanitizing agents used. This will help reduce natural selection for resistant strains of microorganisms within the facility. Multiple sanitizing agents, therefore, should be validated. Environmental monitoring concurrent to use of the manufacturing facility in accordance with established SOPs should be performed to show that the sanitizing program is effective.

4.2.3 Cleaning methods and product changeover

Cleaning method validation is performed primarily to evaluate residual detergent and product levels on washed equipment following use in manufacturing operations. Other testing, such as endotoxin testing, may be included depending on the application of the equipment being cleaned. The effectiveness of the cleaning procedures may be determined by performing assays on the final rinse water that has been processed through the equipment during cleaning or through the use of direct surface testing (i.e., swabs). These assays are used to determine the levels (if any) of residual product or cleaning agent remaining on the equipment after cleaning.

Effective test methods for equipment cleaning procedure validation (as applicable) are visual examination, the Lowry assay for total residual protein level determination, sodium dodecyl sulfate polyacrylamide gel electrophoresis (SDS-PAGE) or immunoassay for product-specific residual protein level determination, total organic carbon assay for residual organic material level determination, limulus amebocyte lysate (LAL) assay for endotoxin level determination, and an ion specific assay (i.e., sodium or phosphate) for residual cleaning agent level determination. The specific test methods and assays chosen will depend upon the equipment configuration, stage in the production process, chemical nature of the product, and the cleaning agent for which the assay is to be performed. A current issue of concern is the sensitivity of the assay in regards to the acceptable level of protein or detergent residue.

4.2.4 Bioinactivation

Bioinactivation of bacterial or cell culture suspension waste or other active processing waste material should be validated. For Biosafety Level 1 Large-Scale (BL1-LS) production using recombinant DNA, the National Institutes of Health (NIH) guidelines [7] require that:

1. Organisms should be inactivated prior to removal from a closed system or other primary containment equipment, and
2. Waste solutions and waste materials should be inactivated, with respect to their biohazard potential.

It is the responsibility of the Institutional Biosafety Committee [7] to define the acceptable level of and methods used for bioinactivation. Typical methods for bioinactivation include heat kill, steam sterilization, and chemical treatment. The bioinactivation process variables (i.e., time, temperature, pH, etc.) should be challenged and monitored and the inactivated materials assayed to measure the effectiveness of the process.

4.2.5 Sterilization methods

The goal of sterilization validation studies is to provide a high degree of assurance that the desired probability of sterility (sterility assurance level) is achieved. Principle sterilization methods include filtration; exposure to steam in an autoclave; steam-in-place (SIP) of process piping, a standing vessel, or a freeze dryer; or heating of a vessel filled with a solution. Validation of a sterilization process can follow either the bioburden approach (based upon lethality calculations) or the overkill approach as described in Parenteral Drug Association (PDA) Technical Monograph No. 1, Validation of Steam Sterilization Cycles [8].

The first task of steam sterilization cycle validation, using the example of an autoclave, is to perform empty chamber heat distribution studies using thermocouples attached to a calibrated data logger. This is done to determine temperature uniformity of the sterilizing medium within the autoclave chamber and to identify the existence and location of any cold spots. Once a manufacturing load has been defined and the sterilization cycle adequately developed, validation of the cycle for a particular load using heat penetration thermocouples and biological indicators (BIs) or direct microbial challenge follows. The challenge microorganisms most often chosen for this purpose are vegetative spores of Bacillus stearothermophilus. The positioning of the thermocouples and BIs within the load are determined during cycle development, with attention focused on identified cold spot(s).

The methods and limitations of the specific BI used must be thoroughly understood prior to performing any cycle development or validation studies. For vendor-supplied BIs, the method required for storage and that used for determining the D-value (BI death rate) may be different from one BI vendor to the next. As an example, one vendor could store his BIs at -20 °C and perform the D-value determination test immediately after removing the BIs from the freezer, while another vendor could require storage of the same type of BI at -20 °C and allow the BI to rest at room temperature for two weeks prior to determining the D-value. These special handling practices are usually printed on the vendor's label claim for the BI. It must be understood that failing to strictly adhere to these same practices during testing could result in a significantly higher (or lower) D-value and possibly jeopardize the validity of the validation study.

4.2.6 Media hold challenge

Often in the processing of sterilized liquid products or intermediates, it is necessary to hold them in a vessel for a period of time and maintain sterility. Both the vessel and the time interval should be challenged to validate the ability of the vessel (piping, valves, filters, etc.) to maintain an adequate barrier to microbiological contamination under defined conditions. Typically, a microbiological growth medium such as trypticase soy broth is sterile filtered into or steam sterilized within the vessel. The medium is held in the vessel under optimal conditions for microbial growth for a time period that equals or exceeds the proposed operating conditions or expiration dating for the manufacturing process. The medium is then inspected for evidence of microbial contamination.

In some cases, such as media hold challenges of bulk processing steps, sterile additions and aseptic manipulations of the medium should be performed during the holding period. Samples of the medium should be taken following the performance of each operation to maintain continuity of the data generated. At the conclusion of the testing, a sample of the medium should be exposed to a microbiological growth promotion test to demonstrate that the medium will support growth.

4.2.7 Depyrogenation

Dry heat is typically used for sterilization and depyrogenation of heat stable materials such as stainless steel or glass. Validation of a depyrogenation process is similar to that for a sterilization process with the exception that an endotoxin challenge is used in place of a BI challenge. This is done because the desired effect of a depyrogenation process is endotoxin destruction. As referenced in Section 6.3.1 of PDA Technical Report No. 3, the times and temperatures typical of overkill depyrogenation processes yield very high spore log reduction (SLR) values and biological challenges, therefore, are not required [9].

Both empty chamber heat distribution studies and loaded chamber heat penetration studies are performed to validate the depyrogenation equipment and process. Cold spot(s) within the exposure chamber or heating zone should be identified during equipment start-up and cycle development and probed during the loaded chamber validation runs. According to the overkill approach to validation of a depyrogenation process, the loaded chamber heat penetration temperature studies must provide assurance that the coolest location within a loading pattern will consistently be exposed to sufficient heat to ensure a minimum of three logs reduction of an endotoxin challenge [9]. Based upon the typical sensitivity and variability of the LAL assay, a recommended starting level for endotoxin challenges would be 25,000 endotoxin units (EU) per challenger container (i.e., vial).

4.2.8 Validation of filtration

Complete validation of a filtration process should include an evaluation of the product, the process step requirements, and the filter medium itself. Filtration will serve different purposes at various steps in the manufacturing process. In the early steps of biochemical manufacturing, filtration may be intended for sterilization of fermentation growth medium, the removal of cellular debris, or diafiltration of the intermediate drug product. Later on in manufacturing, filtration is typically meant to accomplish microbial retention alone without altering the product's composition.

The filter medium must be compatible with the product and give the highest possible yield after filtration. It is therefore important to evaluate more than one type of filter material and to be certain that the appropriate size filter is used. This decision will be based upon the volume of material to be processed and the expected filter loading during filtration of the product, as well as actual yield measurements.

Acceptability of a filter that will be used for microbial retention is determined through the performance of a bacterial challenge test [10] in addition to physical/chemical compatibility testing. When bacterial challenge testing is performed, the actual product that will be filtered should be used for the challenge. This is done because the unique physical and chemical properties of the product may themselves affect the performance of the filter medium [11]. The testing is typically performed by the filter manufacturer using small discs cut from a production lot of filter medium. A copy of the vendor's validation report should be retained by the biopharmaceutical manufacturer. Although most filter manufacturers may provide a wealth of validation data for their products, the user is nonetheless ultimately responsible. This also includes validation of the filter integrity test device used in production.

4.2.9 Programmable logic controllers (PLCs)

The FDA has recognized that computers and computerized systems are an integral part of the wide variety of operations conducted in the pharmaceutical industry and has published a guideline for their field investigators to use when reviewing computerized systems [12]. It has become acceptable practice that the sophisticated computerized systems that control facility environments and production equipment be validated. A clear understanding of the system hardware, software, and the control process must be gained, and the computer's/PLC's operating system (application code) should be documented.

It should be verified that the installation of the computerized system meets the manufacturer's recommendations and design requirements. Furthermore, the operations performed by the system should be documented and challenged through appropriate validation testing [13]. Once a computerized control system has been defined, documented, and validated, change control procedures should be implemented to ensure that the integrity of the system is maintained, and any future changes are properly tested, verified, and documented.

4.3 Validation of bulk drug manufacturing

Validation of bulk drug manufacturing is intended to demonstrate that process controls are adequate to assure consistent product quality. A one-time bulk drug manufacturing validation program should include characterization of the MWCB, testing of product recovery and purification steps, and development of in-process tests. A distinction must be made between validation and routine testing, though both are requirements of GMP. Validation lays the foundation for routine testing such as pre-production screening of the MWCB and in-process testing.

Characterization of the MWCB and screening of each production lot for the presence of contamination by adventitious agents such as bacteria (bacteriophage, in the case of bacterial systems), fungi, mycoplasma, and exogenous viruses are performed to assure the acceptability of the starting cultures for use in production. Process controls are developed and validated to assure that the risks of product contamination or degradation during production and recovery are minimal. Such characterization and process controls apply whether the manufacturing method utilizes production in cell culture or bacterial fermentation.

4.3.1 Characterization of the MWCB

Characterization of the MWCB is performed to provide information that may be used to show that the integrity of the cells and of the DNA remain intact during production, as well as to document the purity of the MWCB. Cell line characterization involves [14,15]:
   1. gathering general information of the history and morphology of the cell line, the plasmid, and its transfection into the host cell;

2. listing the methods used in the storage, maintenance, and propagation of the cell line;
3. determination of cell markers (include banding cytogenics, isoenzyme analysis, and product secretion analysis) relevant to final product purity and cell line identity;
4. tumorigenicity studies;
5. karyology studies;
6. looking for expression of endogenous retroviruses;
7. examining cells from the MWCB for the presence of adventitious agents and other products; and
8. testing the MWCB for the presence of virus, fungi, bacteria, or mycoplasma.

In the case of bacterial production systems, characterization could include, for the host system:

1. carbohydrate utilization,
2. antibiotic resistance,
3. prototrophy/auxotrophy, and
4. contamination;

for the plasmid:

1. sequence and
2. restriction map;

and for the transformed host:

1. growth rate,
2. product expression,
3. plasmid form,
4. plasmid restriction map and sequence, and
5. SDS-PAGE gel product profile.

Testing should be performed to document the stability of the cells and of the genetic materials encoding the product. The PDL of cells achieved during production should not exceed a predetermined upper limit [14]. The growth pattern and morphological appearance of the cells should be shown to be stable to at least 10 PDLs beyond that which would normally be encountered in production.

4.3.2 Recovery and purification

The purpose of product recovery is to separate the drug substance from impurities, contaminants, and process waste that are inherent in the fermentation and other processing of the intermediate product. The ultimate goal is to produce a drug product that meets its predetermined specifications and quality attributes while preventing inadvertent contamination of the product during processing. This is most effectively accomplished by designing, and validating, a production and recovery process that will minimize contamination while maximizing yield.

In biopharmaceutical production, it is often easier to achieve a specific level of product purity than it is to prove it. This is due to a combination of very powerful tools being available for purification of a product and a limited sensitivity for the specific assays that may be used for determining product purity [16]. The goal of validation of product recovery systems and equipment is like that for the validation of equipment cleaning procedures in that we desire to demonstrate that the impurities have been reduced to below predetermined acceptable levels. This applies to all contaminants, whether they be product- or process-related or from extraneous sources. Permissible acceptance limits for foreign materials in the final formulated bulk drug product should be determined to be pharmacologically insignificant in comparison to the activity of the drug substance.

DNA removal from the intermediate product may be effected through the use of ion-exchange chromatography, while virus removal/inactivation may be effected through the use of ultrafiltration, treatment with chaotropes, pH extremes, detergents, heat, chemical derivatization, proteases, conventional separation chromatography, and organic solvents [16]. The specific methods chosen will depend upon the nature of the product, the impurities to be removed, and even the production process itself. Validation of the process for removal of viruses may be used as an alternative to routine product testing for viral or DNA contaminants [17]. Even so, it is encouraged by the FDA that the production process be validated for its ability to eliminate virus or DNA contaminants.

Validation of virus removal/inactivation steps during recovery and purification is intended to document the ability of the process to remove live virus through the use of direct challenges. The degree of virus removal at each step in the process may be considered additive for the purpose of validation of the entire manufacturing process, as long as each virus removal step uses a different mechanism of action (i.e., detergent, pH, and heat). The acceptable log reduction for DNA removal should be based upon the concentration in the process fluid being purified and the maximum specification for the final filled product (i.e., 10 pg/dose).

Scale-down spike recovery studies, identical to the production process, are an effective means of demonstrating viral and DNA inactivation and/or removal. Model viruses are used for such studies because it is impossible to challenge a process with every conceivable virus contaminant. It is therefore a good idea to consider the merits of potential viruses against each other, with consideration for the production environment, raw materials, and host cells, when selecting viruses to be used in these validation studies. Typical viruses used include NIH Rauscher leukemia virus and N2B Xenotropic virus [16].

It should be noted that procedures used to sanitize and regenerate the various resin columns used in recovery and purification should be validated. Also, whatever the product recovery methods chosen, they must be documented and validated through actual physical challenges. A chromatography column that has been exposed to a lot of material for the purpose of product recovery should be decontaminated using validated regeneration procedures prior to reuse of the column [17]. Chromatography column regeneration validation is most frequently accomplished through the use of buffer blank runs, looking for the absence of product to demonstrate the effectiveness of the regeneration process.

4.4 Validation of pharmaceutical manufacturing

The objective of pharmaceutical process validation is to provide documented evidence that a manufacturing process is reproducible and consistently performs as designed. Validation touches upon several topics that overlap manufacturing boundaries, such as cleaning and sterilization. This section discusses validation of the areas unique to the final production stages of pharmaceutical manufacturing (aseptic processing, lyophilization, and packaging). There are several excellent reference texts on pharmaceutical process validation that may be consulted for specifics on designing and implementing a validation program. Two books that are particularly useful are Pharmaceutical Process Validation [18], and Validation of Aseptic Pharmaceutical Processes [19].

4.4.1 Aseptic processing

Validation of aseptic processing is intended to demonstrate that the environment, procedures, and equipment used during all interrelated aspects of aseptic filling of a drug product do not induce contamination of the product. This is typically demonstrated by environmental monitoring, HVAC validation, personnel training and monitoring, and the performance of media fills, which simulate the aseptic filling operation using bacteriological growth medium instead of the drug product [20]. Media fills are supplemental testing that should be used to periodically monitor the total filling environment, equipment, and procedures used for aseptic filling operations, as well as to confirm that significant process or engineering changes in the aseptic processing area are acceptable. Media fills should be performed in accordance with all SOPs and manufacturing formulae used for routine filling operations.

4.4.2 Lyophilization

Lyophilization, or freeze drying, is intended to extend the shelf-life and stability of a product by lowering its moisture content. During lyophilization, a protein-containing solution is first frozen and then subjected to levels of vacuum and temperature that will sublimate the frozen moisture down to a predetermined level. The temperatures, pressures, phase durations, and lyophilized product moisture content are determined through cycle development and stability studies.

During validation, multiple lyophilization cycles are performed using vials containing placebo and active drug to establish the reproducibility of the cycle and the conformance of the lyophilized product to its specifications. Validation of the filling operation must be considered integral to validation of a lyophilization cycle. This is because variations or inconsistency in fill volumes will affect the reconstituted product concentration and the resulting product potency and stability.

4.4.3 Container/closure integrity

The container/closure system is much more than just the combination of components and the method of forming the seal. For a glass vial with a rubber stopper and aluminum cap, the methods for washing and sterilizing the components prior to use cannot be overlooked and must be identical to the actual procedures used during normal manufacturing operations. Whenever possible, the defined limits of the sealing procedures should be challenged.

The task of identifying the variables that affect the quality of a seal often cannot be quantified. We can describe and control the procedures used to prepare the closure components for use, such as the silicone level on washed and siliconized rubber stoppers or the seal force applied by a capping machine. It is, however, more difficult to describe in numbers the various manual adjustments required in the set-up of an automatic capping machine or for a flame ampule sealer. Therefore, every attempt should be made to describe in SOPs, in as much detail as possible, the set-up and operating procedures for the system used to produce the container seal. Once adequate documentation is in place, we can proceed to validate the container/closure system. We must also demonstrate that the integrity of the container seal can be maintained under expected conditions of storage. This is accomplished by challenging the seal under conditions more rigorous than we would expect the product to be exposed to in the field.

There are two readily available test methods for verification of the integrity of the formed container/closure seal: the USP bacterial challenge test and the dye leak challenge test [21]. With suitable assay validation, either method will provide an adequate challenge to the container seal.

4.4.4 Packaging and labeling

Before the product leaves the shipping dock, there should be assurance that the product not only meets its predetermined quality attributes but also that each unit has been properly labelled. The FDA has found that 26–32% of product recalls are due to mislabeling [22]. Label mix-up was noted to be the greatest cause of mislabeling. The most common causes of label mix-ups were found to be the use of undedicated packaging lines, labels that look alike, and the use of cut labels. When these practices are used, extra scrutiny should be required during labelling operations.

The cost of product recall, for any reason, can be devastating to a company. The impact will be not only financial but may be reflected in consumer confidence, the company's reputation, and the overall drug market. Consumer safety and confidence in the drug market are always in question in the face of a product recall.

Validation of labeling is more a matter of choosing the right labels and equipment, operator training, and process flow and control. SOPs for quarantine, inspection, release, and handling of labels, shippers, and product inserts must be in use and effective. The procedures should be simple, logical, and appropriate with respect to the facility layout and product flow through the labeling and packaging area. Some of the most useful practices in preventing labeling mix-ups include 100% machine vision inspection of the labeled product, the use of color coding and size to differentiate products and labels, and the use of bar coding. Additionally, the use of weight checks on the packaging line can be used in identifying missing inserts or product in the final shipper.

Validation of a machine vision system and packaging line weight checker should be performed using limit samples with known defects. These samples may include labels with the wrong lot number or expiration date and packaged product that is missing the product insert or has a product container with a low fill volume.

4.5 General topics

There are several ancillary programs that are required to assure the success of any validation effort. Among these, probably the most important is test equipment and process equipment calibration.

4.5.1 Calibration

Calibration is not intended to be used just for periodically checking gauges, sensors, and switches on production equipment to be sure that they are functioning within process tolerance requirements. In a larger sense, calibration is a useful tool for preventive maintenance and QC of production systems. Likewise, calibration of equipment used for validation is required to assure that it is performing optimally during times of use.

Validation equipment such as data loggers with thermocouples, moisture analyzers, particle counters, and the like, as well as critical process control instrumentation, should be placed on routine calibration programs. Prior to performing any equipment validation, the calibration status of the critical monitoring and controlling instruments associated with the production equipment should be verified, and user standardization should be performed specifically on the instruments that will be used for collecting validation data.

4.6 Conclusion

Validation, in addition to being required by law, is basically good business practice. Through the use of cycle development, validation, training, equipment maintenance, and effective process monitoring and controls, we can assure a high degree of sustained product quality and reduce operating costs. The risk of costly product recalls are minimized, and lot-to-lot product quality and consistency is maximized.

References

[1] *Guideline on General Principles of Process Validation.* May 1987. Division of Manufacturing and Product Quality (HFN-320), Office of Compliance, Center for Drugs and Biologics, Food and Drug Administration, 5600 Fishers Lane, Rockville, MD 20857.

[2] Federal Food, Drug, and Cosmetic Act, Section 501(a)(2)(B).

[3] Title 21, Code of Federal Regulations, Section 210.11. Washington, DC: Office of the Federal Register, National Archives and Records Administration, 1989.

[4] Title 21, Code of Federal Regulations, Section 211.00. Washington, DC: Office of the Federal Register, National Archives and Records Administration, 1989.

[5] Draft Biotech Inspection Outline. Division of Field Investigators (HCF-130), Office of Regional Operations, Office of Regional Affairs, Food and Drug Administration, Aug. 1988.

[6] *USP XXII.* Rockville, MD: The United States Pharmacopeial Convention, Inc.

[7] "Guidelines for Research Involving Recombinant DNA Molecules." Notice. *Federal Register, Part III.* 7 May 1986. Department of Health and Human Services, Office of Recombinant DNA Activities, 12441 Parklawn Drive, Suite 58, Rockville, MD 20882.

[8] *Validation of Steam Sterilization Cycles.* Technical Monograph No. 1. Philadelphia: Parenteral Drug Association, 1978.

[9] *Validation of Dry Heat Processes Used for Sterilization and Depyrogenation.* Technical Report No. 3. Philadelphia: Parenteral Drug Association, 1981.

[10] Howard, G. *Development of a Microbial Challenge Method for the Evaluation of the Retention Characteristics of 0.2 μm-rated Membrane Filters When Filtering High Viscosity Liquids.* Pall Corporation, 1986.

[11] Howard, G. and Duberstien, R. "A Case of Penetration of 0.2 μm-rated Membrane Filters." *Bacteria Journal of the Parenteral Drug Association* (July/Aug. 1978).

[12] *Guide to Inspection of Computerized Systems in Drug Processing.* U.S. Department of Health and Human Services, Public Health Service, Food and Drug Administration, 1983.

[13] Kuzel, N. "Fundamentals of Computer System Validation and Documentation in the Pharmaceutical Industry." *Pharmaceutical Technology* (Sept. 1985).

[14] *Points to Consider in the Characterization of Cell Lines Used to Produce Biologicals.* 1984. Center for Biologics Evaluation and Research (HFB-1), Food and Drug Administration, 8800 Rockville Pike, Bethesda, MD 20892.

[15] Lubiniecki, A. and May, L. "Cell Bank Characterization for Recombinant DNA Mammalian Cell Lines." *Develop. Biol. Standard 60,* (1985):141–146.

[16]   Builder, S.; van Reis, R.; Paoni, N.; and Ogez, J. "Process Development and Regulatory Approval of Tissue-Type Plasminogen Activator" in *Proceedings of the 8th International Biotechnology Symposium.* Paris, 1988.

[17]   *Points to Consider in the Manufacturing and Testing of Monoclonal Anitibody Products for Human Use.* 1987. Center for Biologics Evaluation and Research (HFB-1), Food and Drug Administration, 8800 Rockville Pike, Bethesda, MD 20892.

[18]   Loftus, B. and Nash, R. *Pharmaceutical Process Validation.* New York: Marcel Dekker, 1984.

[19]   Agalloco, J. and Carleton, F. *Validation of Aseptic Pharmaceutical Processes.* New York: Marcel Dekker, 1986.

[20]   *Validation of Aseptic Filling for Solution Drug Products.* Technical Monograph No. 2. Philadelphia: Parenteral Drug Association, 1980.

[21]   *Aspects of Container/Closure Integrity.* Technical Information Bulletin No. 4. Philadelphia: Parenteral Drug Association, 1983.

[22]   Vogel, P. Transcript of speech given by Chief, Non-Sterile Drugs Branch, Office of Compliance, Center for Biologics Evaluation and Research, to International Society of Professional Engineers (ISPE), Bethesda, MD, 15 March 1989.

5 Quality assurance (QA) of production materials for biotechnology

D. H. Miller

Contents

5.1 Introduction

A two-tier system for material selection and control is suggested in most biotechnology organizations: 1. original qualification of the material and 2. lot-to-lot testing for routine release of the material to production. Original qualification consists of initial evaluation and approval for functionality and safety plus generation of specifications and other documentation. This original qualification will be the focus of this chapter.

5.2 QA materials qualification interactions

5.2.1 Research and development (R&D)

QA interactions should start with R&D. In a large organization, it can take considerable time for all R&D personnel to understand that the materials they are using for research are materials about which the QA materials qualification group should know. A high awareness needs to be established that QA materials testing and approval is required for the materials that will be used. R&D needs to contact QA as soon as they have indications a material will be used. If the QA materials qualification group is not involved until development/production starts manufacturing clinical lots, regulatory submissions could be delayed.

5.2.2 Technology

Groups that transfer the process from research through development into production are frequently called technology groups (e.g., manufacturing technology or process development). They do scale-up and move the process into the production area. The QA materials qualification group must be in touch with technology groups because the original process will be changed during the transition. The initial research materials will not always be the materials that work through to production.

5.2.3 Engineering

The engineering department keeps the process operating once a material is in the system. If four different O-rings and diaphragms are qualified for a process and the engineering department doesn't realize that specific materials are required, they may purchase O-rings from random unapproved vendors. They must understand that certain approved materials are required and that they must approve new materials prior to installation. Maintenance and engineering staff will always want to use alternate materials and alternate vendors. This is acceptable as long as they work from a controlled pool of approved vendors and materials.

5.3 Qualification of materials

This review will cover materials qualification from a safety point of view—particularly, evaluation of the amount and toxicity of extractables. Functional qualification must be performed separately by the process research and development engineers.

When materials require safety qualification, the initial step is to generate a qualification request. The requestor states the material to be approved, vendor's identification (including lot numbers), use, process conditions, and other general information needed for evaluation based on the point of use in the process.

A determination of the testing required must be made by the appropriate technical experts. These include, at a minimum, the requestor, the materials safety qualification manager, a chemist, a biologist, and possibly a toxicologist, depending on the material use. Once the needed testing is determined, the tests are run, the results reviewed, and documents generated approving the material for the specific requested use. Subsequent different uses of the same material require additional requests.

If the initial requested lot is for clinical production and it passes all designated tests, the material could be used for production. In this initial, nonroutine production, the QA materials safety qualification manager will have the responsibility of signing off the first few material lots for clinical production. Concurrently, a system of documentation is completed for routine QA release.

5.3.1 Suppliers

It is recommended that small biotechnology companies use the biggest, most experienced, and most technically competent suppliers they can find. It may cost more, but they will be buying expertise to compensate for their lack of internal staff and resources. Most small companies cannot afford and do not have the expertise to do as much raw material testing as is needed. If material is taken on certification from a supplier without proper vendor evaluation, testing, and controls, the company can be assured of problems downstream. There is a series of questions that companies can ask regarding vendors.

5.3.1.1 Responsiveness
Does the supplier meet your timing needs? Does the supplier provide information in a timely manner? Will they notify you if any of their sources of materials change?

5.3.1.2 History
Have you dealt with this supplier before? Do you have a vendor file on the company? Are they known in the industry?

5.3.1.3 Technical knowledge
Can the supplier support the product? Have they been supplying this product for a year or more? Do they have pharmaceutical grade materials and associated documentation? Can they answer all your technical questions now, not after they go to their supplier?

5.3.1.4 Good manufacturing practice (GMP)
Do the suppliers know about GMP and have an understanding of what the product will be used for?

5.3.1.5 Size
A lot of important characteristics are related to the size of the vendor. Your company will receive more support from a larger vendor that will have production capacity, QA, documentation, certificates of analysis, etc.

5.3.1.6   Documentation
Does the vendor have a good specification for the material it is selling? An audit of the vendor should show if the process is under control and whether the vendor can document it.

5.4   Point of use for materials

There are two basic types of uses for materials: nonproduct contact and product contact. There are a lot of nonproduct contact materials in any system that the materials approval group should know about as they proceed. If there is control over materials in the system and that information can be accessed, it helps in solving problems.

5.4.1   Nonproduct contact materials

5.4.1.1   Engineering chemicals
There are many chemicals in this area, and a separate file should be kept on them. The materials qualification group must know about lubricants used on equipment and conveyor belts, coolants used in the manufacturing process including freons and ethylene glycol, cleaning agents used in the facility, materials used in boiler water treatments that frequently contain biocides, and so forth. From time to time, these accidentally find their way into the product. Excellent documentation on composition is very helpful at such times.

5.4.1.2   Sterilants
The primary sterilant used in biotechnology facilities is steam. Water for injection (WFI) is the most desirable water source for sterilant steam. Other water sources may carry over undesirable contaminants such as those from water treatment chemicals. Sodium hypochlorite has been a highly useful sterilant for many years because it is relatively nonhazardous to the handlers. A 500-ppm solution in WFI is a standard concentration for use, but it does attack stainless steel. Some alternates exist (chlorine dioxide types) that claim to be better and less corrosive, but clear evidence of this is not known to the author. Ethylene oxide (EtO) and formaldehyde are now on various carcinogen lists. Hospitals still use them for small sterilization loads. It is very important to "outgas" for at least seven days before using the gas sterilized product to allow the residual toxic materials to defuse out of the product.

5.4.1.3   Pesticides
Pesticides are unacceptable inside GMP facilities. There should not be a pest problem with spraying limited to the exterior perimeter of a tight facility and maintenance of good housekeeping inside. There should be a routine monitoring program. If an infestation occurs where there is no choice but to spray, the production facility has to be brought down, sprayed with a short-acting agent, washed down, and then swabbed and tested for residual pesticide. All activity must be well documented.

5.4.1.4   Paints
Many paints have historically contained lead and mercury compounds, although new paints may not contain these toxic metals. The biggest current problem with paints is the solvents emitted. Total ventilation over a period of several days is necessary to eliminate solvent-based carriers.

5.4.1.5 Packaging

External packaging materials are not critical product safety items. However, containers such as plastic bags that directly contact products should be fully characterized by the product contact methods discussed later.

5.4.1.6 Colorants

Use of colorants is often highly desired by sales and marketing personnel but is acceptable only for nonproduct contact items. The only colorants currently known to the author to have low toxicities are white (titanium or zinc oxides), ultramarine blue, carbon black, and iron oxide red. Most other colorants are based on toxic heavy metals or benzidine-based dyes.

5.4.2 Product Contact Materials

Process materials are high- molecular weight materials that are not intentional components of the product. They may leach low levels of residue into the product but do not intentionally become molecularly intimate with it. Basic chemicals are materials that are put into the product as part of the process. Some of these are normally removed by the time the product is released (e.g., buffers) and some remain with the product (e.g., excipients). Basic chemicals dissolve in the solution and are molecularly intimate with the product.

5.4.2.1 Basic Chemicals

There are two types of basic chemicals for biotechnology purposes: those used in fermentation and those used in purification.

5.4.2.1.1 Fermentation basic chemicals

CELL CULTURE MEDIUM: This dry blend or solution consists mostly of vitamins, amino acids, salts, and biologicals.

WATER: An excellent article on water quality has been written by M.J. Harbage [1]. Water is the primary raw material in all biotechnology processes. The details of assuring water quality are beyond the scope of this chapter. There are anecdotal reports of fermentor failures which cell culture experts have attributed to water quality in the absence of any other explanation. Primary contaminant concerns in water are low molecular weight organics and heavy metals. Water of USP WFI quality is a good starting point for all cell culture quality water.

GASES: Gases can typically be purchased in United States Pharmacopeia (USP) or National Formulary (NF) grades for fermentation.

Use of compendial materials for fermentation is recommended and makes validation of testing unnecessary.

5.4.2.1.2 Purification basic chemicals

These chemicals include primarily buffers, excipients and, of course, injection quality water. Use of USP grade chemicals whenever available for purification is necessary to assure injectable purity of the final product.

5.4.2.2 Process materials (high molecular weight)

There are many high molecular weight process materials, including containers, closures, hoses and piping, affinity antibodies, filters, pumps, gaskets, O-rings, and diaphragms.

5.4.2.2.1   Containers
USP Type I and Type II glass are the best candidates for final containers. If plastics are considered, a major protocol with FDA approval may be required. In some instances, plastics may be used for in-process steps but must be shown not to compromise the product.

5.4.2.2.2   Closures
Elastomeric closures have come to be complex mixtures of materials. Halobutyl compounds with resin cures are showing low extractives and low toxicity. Such discussion is beyond this chapter; however, the reference articles are recommended [2, 3, 5, 8, 10].

5.4.2.2.3   Hoses and piping
If there is a choice, it is recommended that everything with product contact be hard-piped in 300 series stainless steel. If this is not possible from an engineering point of view, flexible hoses may be needed to transfer buffers, product solutions, etc. Production wants a hose that has a wire-mesh braid and is triple-wrapped to allow considerable abuse in the production process.

Although silicone-core hose is the material of choice from an extractables point of view, there are several problems with it. Because of its production process, it can be purchased only in nine- to twelve-foot lengths and is normally reinforced with spiral stainless steel wire and nylon or polyester fabric. If damaged, the steel wire may break and puncture the hose. The hose also has some functional problems with regard to steam and pressure/vacuum flexing over time. Silicone-core hose is excellent from a toxic extractables point of view if it is properly postcured. If this is not done at sufficient time and temperature, cytotoxicity testing will be positive.

The author knows of no high strength hoses available in 50-foot or 100-foot lengths that do not have cytotoxic core materials. Particularly to be avoided are natural rubber and Buna N hoses that are cured with mercaptobenzothiazole, a known toxin and probable carcinogen.

An ethylene propylene diene monomer (EPDM), peroxide-cured hose is the most likely industrial hose candidate. Viton hoses are normally good but very expensive. Vitons are sometimes compounded with lead oxide. These are normally brown rather than black. Teflon is excellent as there are no significant extractives or toxics. It is, however, quite rigid, it cold flows, and it is expensive.

5.4.2.2.4   Affinity antibodies
Affinity antibodies are not intentional components of products. Unfortunately, there is frequently significant leaching of these antibodies from columns to which they are claimed to be covalently bonded. Extensive washing of new columns and antibody monitoring in chromatography solutions and final product are necessary.

If affinity and other chromatography gels are purchased commercially, they will frequently contain low levels of thimerosal or sodium azide. These toxic materials will migrate into the interstices of gel. Rinsing the gel with WFI will not remove all of the components internal to the gel particles. Removal of these toxics is time- and temperature-related. The gel must be soaked (preferably overnight) in WFI, saline, or a buffer solution to allow complete diffusion from the pores. Gels not so treated will exhibit cytotoxicity on extended extraction.

If the gel is only rinsed and not soaked, downstream processes will be contaminated at low levels over extended periods of time. If the nonsoaked gel is used close to the end of the process, low levels of toxic compounds will compromise the product.

5.4.2.2.5 Filters

Filter manufacturers now provide low extractable and low protein binding cartridge and flat stock membranes. To assure that low extractables do not come out of filters into the product, a WFI prewash is always recommended for all pharmaceutical use filters, or validation to show there are no extractables. This wash should be related to surface area and supported by demonstration of removal of residues.

5.4.2.2.6 Pumps

Pumps are not a major issue as peristaltic types are now used in most facilities. Extractables can be found in other types of pumps. If testing of a pump system is desired, sterilize the pump system, take tissue culture fluid (TCF), recirculate it for an extended period of time, then run tissue culture cytotoxicity on the TCF. Additionally, recirculating WFI followed by chemical testing (see testing section) is appropriate to evaluate extractives.

5.4.2.2.7 Gaskets, O-rings, and diaphragms

The most problematic materials for biotechnology process solution contact are those made from rubber. Considerable time and effort can be spent qualifying these materials. Sulfur-based cure systems yield materials unacceptable for pharmaceutical use.

Frequently, the postcure given by the manufacturer on peroxide cured diaphragms is insufficient to drive out peroxide and break down residues. Treating 1/4-inch-thick valve diaphragms four hours at 160 °C only eliminates toxics on the surface. If this diaphragm is cut up and put into a good pharmaceutical extraction medium (e.g., 85% human serum albumin) that has some lipid characteristics, considerable cytotoxicity will be seen. The fluid path surface area in a production facility that is given to diaphragms can be extensive. A typical facility might contain in excess of 1000 diaphragms. A constant flow of low-level toxics can be extracted out of improperly prepared valve diaphragms. Validation of the post-cure process is thus critical.

O-rings are small surface area items. Although the inside edge is the only product contact area, caution and proper pretesting are needed. Avoid purchasing natural rubber, Buna N, and styrene butadiene rubber (SBR) compounds, which are all normally sulfur-cured and will cause toxicity problems. Silicone is the material of choice for O-rings provided no toxic heavy metal fillers are used. Viton is normally an expensive but acceptable second choice. Metals testing is needed to assure the material has not been compounded with lead. Red iron oxide is acceptable.

5.5 Testing

There are two types of USP compendial testing on process materials: plastics [2] and container closure [3] testing. Many materials which pass the USP mouse acute systemic and rabbit intracutaneous tests will not pass cytotoxicity testing. The new USP XXII, in place as of 1 January 1990, specifies a variety of cytotoxicity testing methodologies. The indicated physico-chemical tests are minimal. The limits, when specified, are somewhat high for state-of-the-art materials.

The Japanese Pharmacopeia (JP), European Pharmacopeia (EP) and others are more stringent in some parameters than USP. If a material is intended for non-U. S. markets, the most stringent of the limits must be met. The container closure testing requirements in the JP specifies some tests that are extraordinarily difficult to meet and are not clearly related to product safety. The author

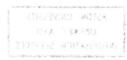

believes that no current U.S. closure will meet them as received. Additional stringent processing and careful initial and lot-to-lot testing will be required to demonstrate compliance with JP.

5.5.1 In-house testing

Well-defined in-house specifications are required for raw materials. These may use USP as a basis; however, additional physicochemical tests on the distilled water extract are recommended and will be discussed later. Input on a case-by-case basis from the toxicology manager, the chemistry manager, and the microbiology manager are necessary. A separate file on each material and documentation of your testing rationale and results are needed.

5.5.1.1 Testing of basic chemicals
Basic chemicals will be molecularly intimate with the product. They are materials which may be dissolved in solutions containing the product, may remain with the product, or be removed from the product. Qualification and routine release tests are listed below.

5.5.1.1.1 Appearance
This is a primary compendial test.

5.5.1.1.2 Identity
This is a primary compendial test. Identity must be performed on all incoming low molecular weight chemicals. Infrared is a good, straightforward test, although some materials do not yield good spectra.

5.5.1.1.3 Assay
This is a primary compendial test. It is necessary to obtain the amount of basic chemical in the sample. High-pressure liquid chromatography (HPLC) is frequently an excellent method. Compendia often use relatively nonspecific wet chemical methods.

5.5.1.1.4 Purity
This is a required compendial test. It is designed to define "impurities". HPLC is frequently the test of choice. Proper validation of the method is important. Thin layer chromatography (TLC) is also a simple, fast test for a variety of basic chemicals, but the quantitation is not as satisfactory as is to be had with a validated HPLC method.

5.5.1.1.5 Toxicity
There are now three primary USP toxicity tests. These include the mouse acute systemic and rabbit intracutaneous tests. These are relatively obsolete.

The in vitro biological reactivity (cytotoxicity) tests in USP XXII provide much better sensitivity than the two animal tests above. Basic chemicals used receive their ultimate cytotoxicity test when they are in the fermentor and in contact with cells. The objective, of course, is to assure nontoxic materials before they are introduced into a large reactor. The recommended test on basic cell culture chemicals is a three-passage cell culture test in growth medium with the organism of use. The reason for running three passages is that the test normally rejects unsatisfactory materials in an acceptable time period. Occasionally, five or more passages are required where serum-based growth factors are absent—from fetal bovine serum, for example.

5.5.1.1.6 Biological purity
These include the issues of pyrogen, virus, mycoplasma, bacterial, and similar contaminations and are beyond the scope of this chapter.

5.5.1.2 Testing of process materials
Process materials are those which contact the product but are not intentionally soluble in it. Extractives are the main issue.

5.5.1.2.1 "As is" testing
IDENTITY: There are several ways of running an identity test on solid high molecular weight materials. Infrared (IR) is reasonably good, unless the material is loaded with carbon black. In this case, pyrolysis-infrared is an alternative.

RESIDUE ON IGNITION (ROI): The solid is ashed at 600 °C. ROI testing gives a semi-quantitative measure of whether or not suppliers are using the same inorganic raw materials they did when the process materials were first qualified. If the ROI changes significantly on subsequent lots of materials, the manufacturer has changed loading or type of filler.

EMISSION SPECTROGRAPHIC ANALYSIS (ESA): Residue on ignition ash is tested for heavy metals. The test will not pick up all toxic elements (e.g., arsenic oxide is too volatile). However, many metals of concern, such as cadmium or lead, will show up. The combined ROI, ESA test is inexpensive and yields considerable information.

5.5.1.2.2 Extracts testing
Distilled water (DW) is the simplest extractant for testing. Other extraction media may contain materials that interfere with the desired tests. For DW extracts, 3000 cm^2 of material surface per liter at 70 °C for 24 hours is the recommended USP condition.

The following tests are recommended on the DW extract:

1. pH for change in acidity from the base line. Limits of 3.5–8.0 are recommended.
2. Oxidizable substances from the USP for purified water is a measure of compounds which will react with potassium permanganate. A limit of not more than 3.0 milliequivalents/ liter (mEq/L) is recommended.
3. USP heavy metals is a rather insensitive test for a number of toxic metals with light-colored sulfides. Not more than 1 ppm is recommended.
4. Buffer capacity from USP is a simple acid/base titration of minimal value.
5. Nonvolatile residue indicates the milligrams (mg) of residue extracted into one liter of DW from 3000 cm^2 surface area. The USP limit is 300 mg; the recommended limit is 50 mg, which no state-of-the-art material should exceed.
6. An ultraviolet scan of the DW extract is recommended as toxic rubber curing agents among others are frequently ultraviolet absorbers.

Toxicity testing is usually done on the DW extract. Historical data with a cell line similar to the USP L-929 line have demonstrated the sensitivity and usefulness of this test. Positive and negative controls are important.

Investigation of DW extracts for pyrogen is definitely justified. Many plastic and rubber materials have been processed in a manner which will destroy pyrogens. There is evidence, however, that it is possible for pyrogens to be adsorbed onto the surface of plastics. Of particular concern for pyrogens is cellulose-based filter media.

Cytotoxicity testing of the process TCF is an excellent way to evaluate a complete piece of equipment such as a fermentor or pump. Recirculation for extended periods of time exacerbates the extraction potential and provides adequate safety factors. Additionally, recirculation of DW followed by the physicochemical tests listed above is recommended.

5.5.1.3 In-process containers

5.5.1.3.1 Stainless steel
300 series stainless steel containers have been used for many years and are satisfactory without further testing. These materials contain 16–26% chromium and 6–22% nickel with the remainder being iron. The most common for pharmaceutical use are 304 and 316. Passivation may be necessary depending on the use. Nickel and chromium are known to be quite toxic in the ionic state. In stainless steel, however, they are bound in the zero state unless oxidation has occurred. No cytotoxicity has been found in DW extracts of high surface-to-volume ratios of 300 series stainless steels.

5.5.1.3.2 Glass
USP Type I borosilicate glass is the accepted standard. If Type II glass is used under USP extraction conditions (70 °C, 3000 cm^2, 24 hours), 400 mg of residue may be extracted, compared to 1–2 mg from Type I glass. The bulk of the extract is soluble silica.

Regulatory agencies have become concerned with aluminum in injectable products due to increasing evidence of toxicity by this route of administration. Type I glass has relatively high levels of aluminum; Type II has lower levels. The article by Victor, et al. discusses this issue [4].

5.5.1.3.3 Plastics
Plastics have many excellent properties as in-process containers. Polypropylene is an excellent material for many uses in contact with TCF. The primary issue is that polypropylene frequently contains antioxidants, which are unnecessary for most biotechnology uses. Polypropylene carboys break down over time under frequent autoclaving and its associated flexing due to cycle pressure changes. Other polymeric materials that normally test satisfactorily for TCF contact include teflon, polyethylene, polysulfone, ethylene vinyl acetate, and silicone.

5.5.1.4 Final containers

5.5.1.4.1 Glass
Glass in final containers raises the same issues that arise in in-process use but with greater urgency. Aluminum is a current issue of concern. Aluminum levels in the product will depend on pH and product characteristics. Beyond standard stability and release testing, aluminum leaching over time must be evaluated.

5.5.1.4.2 Plastics
Materials such as polypropylene are satisfactory in terms of extractables, toxicity, and aluminum levels. A significant concern is with oxygen permeability. There are numerous functional issues

to address. In addition, extensive and expensive extractables and toxicity studies are required to support regulatory submission.

5.5.1.4.3 Bags

A number of pharmaceutical manufacturers use polyvinylchloride (PVC) bags for process solutions and products. The issue is diethylhexylphthalate (DEHP), which is used to plasticize the PVC resin. DEHP is currently on test as a suspected carcinogen. Bags made of ethylene vinyl acetate have excellent potential. Polyethylene bags have various functional problems and frequently contain anti-block and slip agents to improve processing.

5.5.1.4.4 Container closures

State-of-the-art closures are principally made from resin-cured halobutyl polymers. They are generally excellent in terms of extractables and toxicity. White, gray, and black closures are normally acceptable, although some carbon black fillers contain carcinogenic pyrenes and should be evaluated for them. Any other colors demand close testing for heavy metals and toxic/carcinogenic dyes. Container closure safety testing should include at least ROI, ESA, identity by IR, extraction of 3000 cm^2/L surface area in DW for chemistry and toxicology. Toxicology should include USP Class VI and cytotoxicity testing at a minimum. Toxicity testing on extracts made from product solutions are also required. The Parenteral Drug Association's Generic Test Procedures for Container Closures [5] is a useful document outlining recommended lot-to-lot container closure tests.

5.6 Documentation for release of materials

In creating the written documents that QA needs to release materials after the initial validation, it is recommended that individuals from the following departments meet as a committee and be involved in the final documentation generation. The committee should be chaired by the materials safety qualification manager.

PURCHASING should have contact with vendors and send out the requests for vendor audit. Before auditing a vendor, send questions regarding how they control their process and procedures to evaluate whether sending an audit team is justified.

INSPECTION AND RECEIVING must know about new materials. They handle the material on arrival and should be involved in generating the incoming inspection document.

SAFETY AND ENVIRONMENTAL may consider a new material to be hazardous and require that special labels and handling be used. Such safety procedures should be specified on the incoming inspection document.

CHEMISTRY decides tests for initial evaluation and on a lot-to-lot basis. They must develop and validate the tests if they are not compendial.

MICROBIOLOGY decides what initial and lot-to-lot tests are required. A time consuming three-passage (or more) cell culture test may require development and validation.

TOXICOLOGY must recommend validated initial and lot-to-lot toxicity testing as needed.

SPECIFICATIONS must write the product specification which informs the supplier what requirements must be met.

PROJECT ENGINEERING should be available to clearly explain exactly how a material is used in the process.

5.6.1 Documentation needed to operate the materials release system

When material is received, it must have a purchaser's catalog number imprinted by the vendor that refers to a purchase specification agreed to by the supplier. A well-written purchase specification is the basis for returning a product that does not meet requirements.

The QA "Inspection and Release Document", which corresponds to the catalog number, is pulled by the inspector when the material arrives. This document specifies parameters such as color, shape, manufacturer, chemistry testing, biology testing, retain requirements, etc., that must be met and signed off before the material is released for production. This document must reference the specific validated chemistry, biology, functionality, and other written test methods required. Safety and sampling considerations should be specified on the inspection document.

Vendor certifications are sometimes difficult to obtain but frequently are crucial for small companies. Certification may be all that is required on the inspection and release document. It must state test limits and lot results. If a vendor will not supply a high quality certification, purchase the product from a vendor who will. Certifications must be validated periodically by performing tests internally or by contract laboratory to demonstrate test results equivalent to those certified.

Retains are frequently necessary on a lot-to-lot basis. Raw materials for cell culture media may be retained but are not required. If a material is going into the final product, it must be retained per GMP.

5.7 Conclusion

Much progress has been made in the last fifteen years in the understanding and availability of safe and functional materials that will not release extract residues capable of compromising final product or of damaging the single cell organisms so vital to processes in biotechnology. Additional progress is needed in product contact rubber materials. Silicones, if well-postcured, meet the requirements; however, they lack frequently needed functional properties. Peroxide-cured ethylene/propylene rubber, which has good flex resistance, requires well-controlled postcure cycles to remove toxics. Consistent postcure still eludes many manufacturers. Low extractive, nonperoxide-cured rubber products such as the resin-cured halobutyls may offer some solutions.

Rigid plastics such as teflon and polypropylene currently meet industry safety needs when functionality is satisfactory. High quality plastics such as polycarbonates and polymethylpentenes will probably see expanded use.

Stainless steel will continue to be the workhorse product contact material for biotechnology. It must be realized, however, that it is not completely inert and can be affected by a number of process conditions. As a result of this and of cost, high performance plastics will continue to make inroads.

In the long-term, many satisfactory materials for biotechnology use will be available. More important is the understanding by companies in this field of the nature of these materials and the initiation of the quality systems to evaluate and control them.

References

[1]   Harbage, M.J. Quality Systems in Biotechnology-Derived Pharmaceuticals. *American Society for Quality Control, Golden Gate Section* (17 Nov. 1987).

[2]   "Physiochemical Tests—Plastics." *USP XXII* (1990):1572–1573.

[3]   "Elastomeric Closures for Injection." *USP XXII* (1990):1198.

[4]   Victor, R.; Chan, A.K.; and Mattoon, M. "Aluminum Contamination in Albumin Solutions from Glass Storage." *Transfusion 28*(3) (1990):290.

[5]   *Generic Test Procedures for Elastomeric Closures.* Technical Information Bulletin No. 2. Reseearch Committee, Parenteral Drug Association, April 1979.

[6]   Grave, E. "Material Selection for Components in a Pilot Plant Fermentation System." *Biopharm 2* (1988).

[7]   Johnson, H.J.; Northrup, S.J.; et. al. "Biocompatibility Test Procedures for Materials Evaluation *In Vitro."* *Journal of Biomedical Materials Research 19* (1985): 489–508.

[8]   dePoel, W.V. *Developments in Pharmaceutical Rubber Technology.*

[9]   Katz, S.A. "Trace Elements in Biological Tissures and Fluids." *American Biotechnology Laboratories* (March/Apr. 1985):10–17.

[10]   Northrup, S.J. "Cytotoxicity Tests of Plastics and Elastomers." *Pharmacopeial Forum, Stimuli to the Revision Process* (Sept.–Oct. 1984):2939.

[11]   USP Subcommittee on *In Vitro* Toxicity. *Pharmacopeial Forum, Stimuli to the Revision Process* (Jan.–Feb. 1989):4804–4811.

[12]   Miller, W.M.; Lin, A.A.; Wilke, C.B.; and Blanch, H.W. "Polymer Biocompatibility—Effect on Hybridoma Growth and Metabolism." *Biotechnology Letters 8*(7) (1985):463–468.

[13]   "Biological Tests." *USP XXII* (1990):1495–1500.

6 Quality assurance (QA) of analytical methods—biochemical

F. M. Bogdansky

Contents

6.1   Introduction

Biotechnology products include recombinant proteins produced either by fermentation or by cell culture techniques in genetically engineered prokaryotic (bacteria) or eukaryotic (yeast, mammalian cells) systems, and monoclonal antibodies produced from the fusion of spleen cells with a transformed cell line or by the immortalization of lymphocytes by infection with virus. Monoclonal antibodies can be produced either in cell culture or in murine ascitic fluid.

Protein products have the same basic characteristics, and it is these characteristics that require evaluation when developing analytical methods for the routine control of biotechnology products. These characteristics include:

HIGH MOLECULAR WEIGHT: Molecular weights range from 10,000–20,000 Daltons for smaller proteins, such as insulin and interferon, to >950,000 Daltons for IgM monoclonal antibodies.

PRIMARY/SECONDARY/TERTIARY STRUCTURE: Each protein has primary, secondary, and tertiary structure, and all are important in preserving biological activity. Primary structure is defined by the amino acid sequence. Secondary structure is defined by the location of both disulfide bonds and carbohydrate groups. Tertiary structure defines the three dimensional conformation or folding of the protein.

DISULFIDE BONDING: Proteins nearly always have inter- and intra-chain disulfide bonds that are responsible in part for both the molecule's three-dimensional structure and its biological activity.

MULTIPLE CHAINS: Proteins often contain multiple chains, and the correct binding and conformation of these chains is usually critical for biological activity.

CARBOHYDRATE CONTENT: Eukaryotic cells and hybridomas produce glycoproteins. The carbohydrate content and composition of proteins are a consequence of the host organism used for the production of the protein and the conditions under which cell culture is performed.

Biotechnology products have been used in the pharmaceutical and device fields as therapeutic drug products, as *in vivo* diagnostic products, and as *in vitro* diagnostic products. This chapter concentrates on the characterization and control of sterile, injectable biological drug products. The routine control of these biological drug products requires evaluation of the same four parameters used for conventional drug products (i.e., identity, quality, purity, and potency). The major differences lie in the types of tests used, the need for multiple tests to assess a single characteristic, the heavy reliance on the consistency of the manufacturing process to ensure reproducible product, and the use of both end product testing and validation studies to provide assurance that potential contaminants and adventitious agents have been reduced to levels that do not pose a health risk.

A number of important "Points to Consider" documents have been issued by the Food and Drug Administration (FDA) Center for Biologics Evaluation and Research (CBER) to aid manufacturer's in the development of appropriate test procedures and in setting specification limits for the characterization and control of biotechnology protein products [1–4]. These documents serve as an appropriate starting point for individuals involved with the manufacture and control of recombinant proteins and monoclonal antibodies. This chapter intends to present a general overview of analytical methodologies citing the most common practices.

6.2   Physical tests

The routine evaluation of a protein solution's appearance, color, and pH can be used to establish whether or not gross changes have occurred either during the purification process or during storage. The formation of particles in protein solutions is often a serious problem, especially for large proteins that are known to aggregate or for highly unstable proteins, particularly if they are formulated in buffer solutions at a pH close to the protein's isoelectric point. These proteins can be denatured at air/liquid interfaces or by shear effects, and this denaturation often leads to protein precipitation. Stabilizers, including sugars and/or surfactants, are frequently included in final formulations to prevent or minimize denaturation and precipitation.

The quantitation of particulates in solution by liquid particle counting methods can provide important information on the stability of the protein during process and formulation development studies and during storage. Procedures and criteria, such as those described in USP, Chapter <788>, "Particulate Matter in Injections" [5], can be used as a starting point for establishing appropriate criteria for particulates in protein solutions.

6.3   Identity tests

The identity of a protein product is typically established by a combination of several test methods since no single method provides definitive identification. These identity tests can include: 1. determining the molecular weight of both the intact molecule and any subcomponents using sodium dodecyl sulfate polyacrylamide gel electrophoresis (SDS-PAGE) or size exclusion high-performance liquid chromatography (HPLC) procedures, 2. measuring retention times in HPLC assay systems, 3. comparing isoelectric focusing patterns with those of known reference materials, 4. reaction with specific antibody reagents, 5. performing partial N-terminal and C-terminal sequence analysis, and 6. confirming the ability of the sample to demonstrate biological activity in either *in vitro* or *in vivo* assays. More recently, peptide mapping has emerged as a highly accurate identity test for biological products that approaches the specificity of the infrared (IR) spectral analysis used for chemical drug products.

6.3.1   Polyacrylamide gel electrophoresis (PAGE)

Electrophoresis describes the migration of charged particles in an electric field. In stabilizing media such as polyacrylamide gel, the pore size of the gel approaches the dimensions of protein molecules, and molecular sieving as well as molecular charge produces separation of even closely related proteins. In general, 5% acrylamide gels provide separation of proteins with high molecular weights of 90,000 to 750,000 daltons, 7.5% gels are most frequently used for proteins in the molecular weight range of 30,000 to 150,000 daltons, and 12.5% gels are used for the separation of smaller proteins and peptides of 10,000 to 90,000 daltons. Gradient gels, such as a 3–7.5% or 10–27% gradient, can be used when a broader spectrum of molecular weight species needs to be resolved.

Following electrophoresis, the separated protein bands may be visualized with different types of protein-reactive stains. The most commonly used stains are Coomassie blue and silver nitrate. Greater sensitivity is achieved with the silver stain ,which may be employed when detection of very low levels of protein species is critical. Poor specificity of the silver stain makes quantitation of protein mixtures, especially glycoproteins, difficult. In the presence of sodium dodecyl sulfate, an inverse linear relationship between migration distance and the log of a protein's molecular weight has been found. The molecular weight of the intact protein, therefore, can be determined from SDS-PAGE gels run under nonreducing conditions. When the protein is treated with sodium dodecyl sulfate and a reducing agent such as 2-mercaptoethanol, inter- and intra-molecular disulfide bonds are dissociated and the molecule is broken down into its individual subcomponent protein chains. The molecular weight of these subcomponent species can then be determined from the reduced SDS-PAGE gel.

6.3.2 Isoelectric focusing

Isoelectric focusing (IEF) is based on the migration of a protein through a pH gradient in the presence of an electric field. The protein stops migrating and is focused at the point where the pH of the gradient is equal to the protein's isoelectric point (pI) (i.e., the pH where the protein has no net charge). pH gradients are established in agarose or polyacrylamide gels by ampholyte molecules that migrate to their own isoelectric points in an electric field. Following focusing, proteins are visualized by staining with Coomassie blue or silver nitrate and the isoelectric points determined by direct measurement using a surface electrode; by cutting out zones of gel, eluting the protein, and measuring its pH; or more typically by the use of pI marker proteins.

Isoelectric focusing can be very effective in identifying subtle changes in a protein's amino acid composition and sequence, as well as in the carbohydrate content of the purified protein. The isoelectric banding pattern, therefore, is not only an effective identity test but is also effective in identifying changes in the protein due to oxidation or deamidation at selected amino acid residues.

6.3.3 Sequence analysis

Partial N-terminal and C-terminal sequence analysis through 15–20 residues is used to confirm the primary structure of recombinant proteins and monoclonal antibodies and, therefore, serves as an identity test. N-terminal sequence analysis is performed by carrying out sequential Edman degradation of the protein and identifying the resulting amino acids by HPLC [5]. Phenylisothiocyanate reacts quantitatively with the N-terminal amino acid to yield a phenylthiocarbamylamino acid derivative that is cleaved from the protein with trifluoroacetic acid, exposing the next N-terminal amino acid. The cleaved, derivatized amino acid is converted to a phenylthiohydantoin (PTH) amino acid that is isolated and quantitated by reverse phase HPLC. Sequence analysis is typically performed using automated commercial sequencers. C-terminal sequence analysis is performed by cleaving the C-terminal amino acid either with carboxypeptidase enzymes or by reaction with chemicals such as hydrazine or cyanogen bromide.

6.3.4 Peptide mapping

When a protein is subjected to limited proteolysis with enzymes such as trypsin, chymotrypsin or thermolysin, cleavage occurs at defined locations along the backbone of the molecule, giving rise to a known number of peptide fragments of fixed composition. These fragments can be separated by ion exchange or reverse phase HPLC, by SDS-PAGE, or by capillary electrophoresis. HPLC is generally used to separate fragments produced from the digestion of smaller proteins (less than 100,000 mol. wt.), while electrophoresis is applied to the separation of fragments formed from the digestion of antibodies and other large molecular weight proteins.

The digestion pattern produced by each enzyme is unique for each protein; therefore, peptide mapping can be used to confirm the identity of the protein. Because the sites for enzyme digestion are dependent both on the primary structure (amino acid sequence) and on the secondary structure (carbohydrate content and disulfide bonds) of the protein, peptide maps can be used to detect incorrect disulfide binding and changes in the carbohydrate content of the protein. Small changes in the molecular structure such as single amino acid substitutions may be detected by this relatively sensitive method. The reproducibility of the enzyme map is dependent on the purity of the enzyme preparations used and on the consistency of the digestion procedure. In addition, the interpretation of enzyme maps is complex since there may be multiple explanations for a single change. However, differences in the mapping pattern among multiple lots of a single protein can be an indicator of degradation or of a subtle change in the manufacturing process.

6.4   Assays

A variety of assays are used to quantify proteins, including assays to measure total protein content, intact protein, amino acid composition, degradation species, and the carbohydrate content of glycosylated proteins. These assays are used to evaluate lot-to-lot consistency of the drug product and to monitor the stability of the product with time.

6.4.1   Total protein assays

Protein measurements can be made by a variety of colorimetric methods including the Lowry, Biuret, Bradford, and bicinchoninic acid (BCA) assays. These assays measure total protein and, therefore, are not specific or stability indicating. In addition, each requires an external reference standard for protein quantitation. The Lowry procedure uses Folin-Phenol Reagent and involves reaction of the protein with copper (II) in alkali followed by the reduction of phosphomolybdic/ phosphotungstic reagent by tyrosine and tryptophan residues present in the molecule to produce a blue color. The Biuret reaction produces a purple color resulting from the formation of a coordination complex between copper (II) ions and four nitrogen atoms of peptide bonds in the protein. The Bradford assay employs binding of Coomassie brilliant blue dye to the protein and measuring the absorbance of the blue protein-dye complex. The BCA assay involves reaction of the protein with BCA to produce a blue color.

In each of these protein assays, quantitation is made from absorbance measurements by interpolation from a standard curve. Bovine serum albumin and human serum albumin often are employed as reference standards, since they can be obtained in high purity and are stable. However, purified samples of the actual protein product provide the best reference standard, since the intensity of the color response in each of these assays depends on the composition of the individual protein.

Protein content also can be determined directly from absorbance measurements at 280 nm, provided the extinction coefficient of the protein is known and the protein has been shown to be pure by methods such as SDS-PAGE and HPLC and free of contaminants and/or additives that absorb at 280 nm. Extinction coefficients can be determined from dry weight measurements or from spectrophotometric measurements at 205 nm, 235 nm, and 280 nm using the procedures described by Scopes [6] and by Whitaker and Granum [7]. Once the extinction coefficient is known, absorbance at 280 nm provides a very accurate measure of protein content because no reference standard is required and no manipulations other than sample dilution are required. For accurate measurement, care must be taken to assure complete solubility of the protein in the buffer of choice. The Lowry procedure is 10–20 times more sensitive than measurements at 280 nm and 100 times more sensitive than the Biuret and Bradford methods, but the reaction is subject to interference from a number of substances including phenols and serum constituents. Both the Biuret and the BCA assays are less subject to interference than the Lowry assay. The UV assay is subject to interference from nonprotein UV-absorbing contaminants.

Total nitrogen measurement also may be used in place of colorimetric assays, especially for in-process needs. Kjeldhal or, more efficiently, the use of a nitrogen analyzer may be used to obtain total nitrogen content. This information, combined with the known nitrogen composition of a molecule of the protein, will yield an accurate total protein measurement.

6.4.2 Native protein

Numerous degradation mechanisms can result in a protein that has been altered from its natural, native form. These include fragmentation, aggregation, denaturation (i.e., loss of conformation), and chemical modification of constituent amino acids and/or carbohydrate groups. These mechanisms may occur singly or in combination, and all represent degradation of the protein. The principle route(s) of degradation can often be identified by subjecting the protein to elevated temperatures, although caution is required in performing this extrapolation since the degradation mechanism found at elevated temperatures may not be the same mechanism that is followed under normal storage conditions.

Proteolytic and/or hydrolytic degradation is characterized by fragment formation. Depending on the relative location of the cleavage site and the site(s) required for biological activity, fragments may retain biological activity, or the degradation may destroy activity. In some cases, proteolytic or hydrolytic cleavage gives rise to "nicked" molecules in which the fragments are held together by disulfide bonds. Under nonreducing conditions, these nicked molecules cannot be distinguished from native protein. However, in the presence of a reducing agent, the disulfide bonds are reduced and the fragments formed by the cleavage released.

The formation of aggregates can also be a major degradation route for proteins. Native, monomeric proteins can form dimers, trimers, or other higher molecular weight aggregates, which may coalesce to form insoluble precipitated protein. Aggregates may retain biological activity, or aggregation may result in denaturation and a loss of potency.

Size exclusion, ion exchange, and reverse phase HPLC and SDS-PAGE are effective in separating degraded and aggregated protein from native protein. Fragments are easily visualized on reduced and nonreduced SDS-PAGE gels and can be quantitated by densitometry following staining of the gels with Coomassie blue. Aggregates often are seen in reverse phase or ion exchange HPLC as shifts in retention time or as peak broadening. In general, size exclusion HPLC is effective in resolving aggregates from monomeric protein, although resolution is often incomplete. SDS-PAGE also can be used to separate aggregate from native protein unless the aggregate population becomes heterogeneous with respect to molecular weight.

In general, SDS-PAGE provides good resolution of molecules with similar molecular weights and resolution of species over a broad molecular weight range. Relative quantitation of resolved species can be made by densitometry following protein staining. HPLC assays also provide important information about the homogeneity of protein preparations, although typically two or more different types of HPLC are required to confirm the proteins basic structure.

Denaturation of the native protein can occur by physical manipulation of the protein (i.e., by shaking, filtration, or treatment with organic solvents) and, most critically, may result in loss of biological activity. This event may be detected as a loss of activity in a potency assay, provided the denaturation is severe enough and the bioassay is sufficiently sensitive and reliable. Denaturation also can be evidenced by the formation of precipitated protein.

The chemical modification of native protein commonly, but not exclusively, results from oxidation and/or deamidation of individual amino acid residues in the molecule. Depending on the extent of the degradation, these changes can be detected by the potency assay if the change has occurred at the active site or by amino acid sequence analysis. Sequence analysis is particularly effective in detecting changes to the N-terminal amino acid. Peptide mapping and IEF may also be sensitive to subtle changes in the protein.

6.4.3 Amino acid composition analysis

Amino acid analysis is used to quantitate the amount of each amino acid in a protein. The amino acid composition can be used to establish protein identity by comparing the amino acid ratios of test samples with theoretical values determined from the gene structure or with values obtained from the careful analysis of reference standards. For small proteins and peptides, amino acid analysis also can be used to evaluate purity, provided nearly integer ratios can be obtained for the amino acids. Amino acid analysis can be a routine control test, but more often it is used for the characterization of the purified protein following a change in the manufacturing process or for the characterization of a reference standard.

Amino acid analysis is performed by first digesting the protein with acid into its amino acid components. This usually requires multiple hydrolyses under various conditions to produce complete cleavage and recovery of all amino acids. The resulting amino acids can be quantitated by ion exchange column chromatography followed by postcolumn derivatization with ninhydrin; by reverse phase HPLC with precolumn fluorescent derivatization of primary amino acids with OPA (o-phthaldialdehyde) and secondary amino acids with NBD (4-chloro-7-nitrobenzofurazan) or FMOC (9-fluorenylmethyl-chloroformate); or by reverse phase HPLC with postcolumn derivatization using fluorescamine or OPA.

Each method has its particular advantages and disadvantages. Precolumn derivatization provides high selectivity and sensitivity, but low responses are obtained with certain amino acids (cysteine, lysine, hydroxylysine and secondary amino acids) and the derivatized amino acids are unstable, which leads to poor reproducibility. Postcolumn derivatization methods that use fluorogenic reagents provide high sensitivity but require specialized instrumentation and have poorer reproducibility due to the instability of the fluorescent derivatives. Classical ion exchange chromatography followed by colorimetric derivatization using ninhydrin provides reliable amino acid determinations when sample size is not a consideration.

6.4.4 Carbohydrate content analysis

Recombinant proteins produced in bacteria are not glycosylated. However, monoclonal antibodies and recombinant proteins produced by eukaryotic cells are usually glycoproteins, and the extent of glycosylation is dependent on the cell line used for the production of the protein and the conditions under which the protein is produced. The sugars commonly found in glycosylated proteins include fucose, galactose, glucose, mannose, xylose, N-acetyl-glucosamine, N-acetyl-galactosamine, and sialic acid.

Total carbohydrate content is determined by reaction with phenolsulfuric acid followed by quantitation from absorbance measurements at 490 nm. Following acid hydrolysis, quantitation of individual sugars is performed by either ion exchange HPLC or by gas chromatography. More recently, methods are available that permit the cleavage of intact oligosaccharide side chains with endo- and exoglycosidases. The sugar chains then can be identified and quantitated by ion chromatography.

6.4.5 Immunoassays

Assays employing specific antibodies to the protein product may be used in conjunction with total protein measurements to determine specific activity (activity/mg protein). Radio immuno-assays (RIA), immunoradiometric assays (IRMA) and enzyme-linked immunoassays (EIA and ELISA) are examples of commonly used immunoassays. IRMA and ELISA use an antigen or antibody bound to a solid phase upon which a "sandwich" of second antibody and antigen is built (see section 6.5.1). RIA involves competition binding of a specific antibody for both a known amount of radio-labeled protein and an unknown amount of unlabeled protein. The amount of inhibition of binding to the labeled protein is directly correlated to the concentration of protein in the sample.

6.5 Purity tests

The purity of biotechnology products is affected by protein contaminants and degradation products that co-purify with the protein or form during processing and by impurities introduced with the starting materials or during the purification process. The starting materials, including the manufacturer's working cell bank and raw materials used for cell culture or fermentation, can be the source of contaminants such as mycoplasma, bacteria, mold and yeast, bacterial endotoxins, adventitious virus, host cell DNA, host cell proteins, and added chemicals, including antifoams, antibiotics, and inducing agents.

Purification processes for biotechnology products are usually centered around column separation procedures and often include affinity chromatography steps that either provide primary purification of the protein or are included to remove specific contaminants. Since the chemical linkage between an affinity ligand and the solid support is potentially labile, affinity ligands can leach from the chromatography columns and become contaminants in the purified protein. Columns that are used repeatedly for protein purification are a potential source of both microbial contamination and bacterial endotoxins. In addition, chemicals can be added throughout the purification process, and the absence of these added chemicals in the final product must be demonstrated. These added chemicals can include agents used for cleaning processing equipment, agents and preservatives used for the cleaning and storage of separation columns, and ingredients contained in buffers used in the purification process but that are not desirable in the final product.

The absence of process contaminants and degradation products in the final product is demonstrated by a combination of final product testing and process validation studies. A partial list of potential process impurities and the analytical technique used for their detection and quantitation is presented in Table 6.1. Each category is described in more detail in the following sections.

Table 6.1 Potential contaminants in biotechnology-derived proteins

Potential Contaminants	Test Method	Sensitivity
Starting Materials		
Protein Contaminants	SDS-PAGE	0.2–1%
	EIA/RIA	1–500 ppm
Added Chemicals	GC, HPLC, NMR, AA, EIA Wet Chemistry	1 ppm–0.1%
DNA	Hybridization Analysis	1–5 pg
Mycoplasma —cultivable	Agar/Broth Culture	10 CFU/mL
—noncultivable	Co-Cultivation with Vero Cells	100 CFU/100 mL
Bacterial Contaminants	Agar Plate-Count	1 CFU
Bacterial Endotoxins	Limulus Lysate Assay	0.03 EU/mL
Adventitious Agents —viruses	Cell Culture/Focus and Plaque Formation	5–100 PFU/mL or 5-100 FFU/mL
Purification Process		
Affinity Ligands	EIA/RIA	1–500 ppm
Added Chemicals	GC, HPLC, NMR, AA, EIA Wet Chemistry	1 ppm–0.1%
Bacterial Contaminants	Agar Plate-Count	1 CFU
Bacterial Endotoxins	Limulus Lysate Assay	0.03 EU/mL

6.5.1   Protein contaminants

The detection and quantitation of protein contaminants and degradation products that may co-purify with the protein of interest require the development of sensitive and specific assays. SDS-PAGE run under both reducing and nonreducing conditions provides a very effective method of separating unknown protein impurities and degradation products from intact protein. Following electrophoresis, resolved impurity bands can be visualized by staining with Coomassie blue. The visualized bands can then be quantitated by densitometry and area normalization or by densitometry and interpolation from a standard curve. Since different proteins have different Coomassie blue staining affinities, the accuracy of the quantitation is dependent on a knowledge of the staining intensity of each impurity and degradation product. Efforts should be made to isolate and identify contaminants and degradation products. Once isolated and characterized, these impurities and degradation products can be used as reference standards during assay validation studies.

In general, SDS-PAGE with Coomassie blue staining has a sensitivity of 0.2–1%, depending on the protein, and provided that this level of impurity is represented in a single resolved band. The quantitative power of this analytical method is limited when multiple diffuse bands are present. Sensitivity can be increased by visualizing the resolved bands with silver nitrate. Silver binds to the proteins, producing a black band, but the binding is not stoichiometric. Silver staining is usually 10–100 times more sensitive than Coomassie blue staining, although the increase in sensitivity varies from protein to protein. Quantitation of silver-stained gels is usually not possible because the band intensity response is not linear, especially when carbohydrate is present, and because high background staining is frequently found.

Care must be exercised in quantitating degradation products from SDS-PAGE gels to avoid overestimating the total degradation. An understanding of the degradation pathway is essential so that the origin of multiple species can be established. For example, a single cleavage may give rise to two or more fragments; therefore, the extent of degradation cannot be determined as the arithmetic sum of the amount of each fragment.

The detection of protein impurities at levels below 0.1–0.5% typically requires an enzyme immunoassay or a radioimmunoassay that has been developed to detect a specific contaminant. The assay and the assay reagents are customized to the product's manufacturing process. The ability of the test to provide reproducible results is dependent on the lot-to-lot uniformity of the reagents. These immunoassay reagents typically have sensitivities in the range of 1–100 ppm.

ELISAs are frequently employed for quantitating impurities at the ppm level. In these procedures, either an antigen or an antibody against the impurity of interest is immobilized onto a microtiter plate. The test article is added to the wells of the plate so that the potential contaminant can bind to the immobilized antigen or antibody. Following this reaction, a second antibody reagent, consisting of a detector (i.e., an enzyme or a fluorescent tag bound to an anti-impurity antibody) is added to the plate. The second antibody binds to the immobilized impurity, forming a sandwich with the impurity bound between the two test reagents. Quantitation of the amount of bound impurity is made by reacting the second antibody reagent with a specific substrate to produce either fluorescence or a colored solution whose absorbance can be measured spectrophotometrically. Quantitation is then made by interpolation from a standard curve. For these assays to be truly effective in accurately quantitating impurities, the impurities must be isolated and characterized so that they can be used in reagent preparation and as reference standards in the assays.

6.5.2 Added chemicals

Fermentation, cell culture, and protein purification processes commonly require the addition of various chemicals to aid in fermentation or cell culture, to perform specific separation functions, or to protect against destruction of the protein during purification. The absence of these chemicals in the final product can be demonstrated by end-product testing and by validation studies that quantitate that the process is effective in eliminating these added substances.

Since these added substances are primarily chemicals, a wide variety of sensitive analytical methods, including gas chromatography, atomic absorption spectroscopy, NMR, HPLC, immunoassay, and bioassay, can be employed for final product testing. Expectations are that these added chemicals will be removed to levels near or below the detection limit of the assay. Validation studies employing radio-labeled chemicals are conducted on a small scale to measure removal of each added substance by individual steps in the process. Studies also are conducted during manufacturing runs to quantitate removal at each processing step to confirm by mass balance calculations the complete clearance of these added substances.

6.5.3 Affinity ligands

Purification procedures for recombinant proteins and monoclonal antibodies often include passing the material over an affinity column to achieve a high (>90%) degree of purification in a single step or to remove a defined contaminant. The affinity media usually consists of a monoclonal or polyclonal IgG immunoglobulin or a large protein antigen bound to a solid support through a chemical linkage.

Since these linkages may be labile, the protein or antibody may leach from the support and become a contaminant in the protein being purified. Since these contaminating proteins are highly undesirable in the purified product, end-product testing must be able to detect the affinity ligand at the ppm level, and immunoassays are typically employed. Depending on the nature of the affinity ligand, reagents for these assays can either be obtained from commercial sources or produced and quality controlled in-house. In addition to end-product testing, validation studies showing that purification steps downstream of the affinity chromatography step remove the affinity ligand provide strong supporting data that the final protein product is free of the potential contaminant.

6.5.4 Residual DNA

Concern continues to exist regarding the presence of DNA in purified biotechnology products, since these proteins are derived from transformed cell lines or from genetically altered host organisms. Host cell DNA is found in the starting material (i.e., the fermentation paste, the fermentation supernatant, or the cell culture fluid) and arises from dead and lysed cells. The purification process must be designed to reduce host cell DNA to very low levels, and the extent of the removal should be confirmed by both validation studies and end product testing.

Residual host cell DNA in purified proteins can be quantitated by a DNA hybridization assay using a radio-labeled probe prepared by nick translation of DNA extracted from the host cell or from the transformed cell line. Sample DNA is separated from the protein by extracting the DNA with phenol and then precipitating any remaining protein with alcohol. The DNA is denatured with heat, and the single-stranded DNA is immobilized on nitrocellulose membranes. Following hybridization and autoradiography, residual DNA is quantitated by visual comparison to a series of standards. Although DNA content in biological drug products is evaluated on a case-by-case basis, FDA (CBER) guidelines require the DNA assay to have a sensitivity on the order of 10 picograms DNA per dose (1–3), and the World Health Organization (WHO) guidelines require less than 100 picograms per dose [8].

6.5.5 Bioburden and bacterial endotoxins

Since most therapeutic biotechnology products are administered parenterally, the purified protein must be free of bacterial endotoxins and other pyrogenic substances. Bacterial endotoxins in protein products can be quantitated using the limulus amebocyte lysate (LAL) assay. Lysates with sensitivities of 0.03 EU/mL are recommended for use with protein products [9]. The rabbit pyrogen test as described in 21 CFR 610.13(b) [10] and in USP, Chapter <151>, "Pyrogen Test", is used for end-product testing to ensure freedom from pyrogenic substances.

The validation of the removal of bacterial endotoxins from the starting materials by the purification process can be demonstrated on a small scale by spiking column loads and process intermediates with endotoxin and quantitating clearance, or on a production scale by monitoring endotoxin clearance at each process step and verifying overall clearance by mass balance calculations.

6.5.6 Cultivable and noncultivable mycoplasma

Since both recombinant proteins and monoclonal antibodies are produced by cell culture methods, it is possible that the cell culture fluid can become contaminated with mycoplasma. The absence of mycoplasma in the purified protein must be demonstrated by end-product testing, and the purification procedure must be validated to demonstrate the clearance of mycoplasma. The absence of cultivable mycoplasma in the purified protein can be demonstrated by broth and agar culture under both aerobic and anaerobic conditions using the procedure described by CBER [2]. Freedom from noncultivable mycoplasma can be demonstrated by bisbenzimidazole fluoro-chrome staining following incubation of the test sample with Vero cells [2]. A preference for testing unfiltered and quick-frozen/single-thaw samples has been recently expressed by CBER.

Validation studies can be used to support periodic rather than lot-by-lot testing for myco-plasma. These studies involve the spiking of starting materials and/or column load materials with high titers of mycoplasma, simulating the purification steps on a small scale, and calculating mycoplasma removal/inactivation factors. Purification processes should show the clearance (inactivation plus removal) of at least six logs of mycoplasma.

6.5.7 Adventitious agents

An area of great concern at the present time is demonstrating that the purified protein is free of adventitious agents, especially viruses. This must be demonstrated by both end-product testing and by validation data that show the removal of viruses to levels that no longer present a risk factor. The assessment of risk is evaluated on a case-by-case basis and is based in part on the patient population, on the dose level and regimen, and on the health status of the patients.

The identification and quantitation of viral particles in the master cell bank (MCB) and the manufacturer's working cell bank (MWCB), and the identification of infectious virus produced by the MCB and the MWCB are of primary importance. Viral particle enumeration in the MCB/MWCB can be accomplished by thin section electron microscopy, although the sensitivity of this method is 10^6–10^8 particles/mL. Infectious retrovirus can be detected by reverse transcriptase testing, direct assay, or co-cultivation of MCB/MWCB cells with detector cell lines known to support the replication of viruses.

If infectious virus can be detected, then end-product testing for those virus(es) can be performed using an appropriate *in vitro* cell-based plaque or focus assay. Viral assays that first employ amplification of the virus and then detection in a cell culture system are more sensitive than direct cell culture assays and thereby provide greater assurance of the absence of infectious virus.

Validation studies are needed to demonstrate the removal and inactivation of virus by column purification steps and by processes and/or formulations that are designed specifically to inactivate virus. If infectious viruses have been identified, they can be used in small-scale studies to measure clearance and inactivation. Similarly, radio-labeled viral particles prepared by culturing the MWCB in media containing radiolabeled nutrients can be used to measure and define particle removal. Typically, logs of viral clearance (inactivation plus removal) are expected for processes used for the purification of a biotechnology protein product.

6.6   Potency tests

Routine potency testing is unique to biological products. These potency tests measure the dose-dependent biological activity of the intact molecule and demonstrate that the primary, secondary, and tertiary structure of the protein was preserved during production and purification processes. Potency tests are designed to mimic the *in vivo* activity or function of the biological product.

Potency tests can be performed in animals, in *in vitro* cellular assays designed to simulate *in vivo* activity, or in cell-free *in vitro* systems where the assay is designed to reproduce a biological property of the protein—for example, binding to a specific antigen as measured by an ELISA method. Where possible, *in vitro* cell culture assays are preferred over assays that require animals because of the large variability and poor precision of assays that require the use of animals. In general, cell-free potency assays are less desirable than those employing a living system. Examples of potency assays include measuring:

1. protection of cells/animals from viral infection,
2. clot dissolving properties,
3. binding of antibodies to cells containing specific antigens,
4. increases in weights of hypophysectomized animals,
5. inhibition of protein synthesis in cellular or cell-free systems, and
6. inhibition of DNA replication in a target cell system.

Wherever possible, potency measurements should be correlated to international (WHO) or other recognized natural reference standards (NIH, USP) and expressed as international (IU), NIH, or USP units. Potency tests may or may not be stability-indicating, since degradation products may or may not have activity similar to or identical with the biological activity of the intact molecule. The activity usually depends on the relative locations of the biologically active site(s) in the intact molecule and the nature and location of the modification that has occurred to the intact molecule during degradation. If the potency assay is not stability-indicating, an alternate assay, usually SDS-PAGE or HPLC, must be used to measure degradation and/or aggregation of the protein.

Reagent consistency is essential in maintaining a reliable potency assay that provides comparable results from week to week and from assay to assay. The maintenance and passage of the test cell line must be carefully monitored. Lot-to-lot evaluation of growth media and growth media supplements, including fetal bovine serum, must be performed and suitable acceptance criteria established for each individual component. Potency assays require well-characterized in-house reference standards for use in quantitation and well-characterized controls to establish the acceptability of individual assays. Potency assays are usually complex, and, because of the need for extended and multiple incubation times, they usually require multiple days to complete. System precision often can lie in the 30–40% range, and numerous replicates and extremely tight control of reagents and test procedures are needed to reduce precision to the 15–25% range. Frequently, assays are run in at least triplicate on two or more days by two or more analysts to obtain a potency value within a satisfactory confidence interval.

6.7 Conclusion

Although not unique to biotechnology products, the need for process validation as a component of the quality control of biotech products is critical. Because of the complex nature of protein molecules, end-product testing alone is insufficient in detecting subtle changes in these large molecules. At best, these routine tests serve as indicators that the process has remained under control. The process and the careful definition of process variables are responsible for product quality, and consistent, acceptable quality is a result of manufacturing steps that are performed in a reproducible manner time after time. Subtle or uncontrolled changes in a manufacturing process can be responsible for significant changes in a product's purity profile or in the actual structure of the protein.

Early characterization and validation of the manufacturing process for biotechnology products are required. Since column chromatography steps serve as the central downstream purification procedures, an understanding and definition of the function of each chromatography step must be generated. In fact, by knowing the performance capabilities of each processing step, a determination can be made that the process is capable of reducing impurities below established levels. The acceptable levels for potential contaminants are derived on a case-by-case basis and are based in part on the patient population, the dose regimen, and health/safety risk to patients receiving the drug product. By reviewing these factors, determinations can be made as to whether the purification process contains a sufficient number of steps or the most effective steps to achieve the desired reduction in the level of impurities. Process validation demonstrates early on whether the process is reproducible.

Biotechnology products are complex, their routine quality control testing is complex, and the consistent quality of the product is derived from a well-defined manufacturing process performed in a reproducible and controlled manner as verified using validated assays. The product's identity, strength, quality, and purity are established from a combination of test procedures which, when taken together, confirm that the manufacturing process has been effective in producing an acceptable product of high and consistent quality whose biological activity has been preserved throughout the processing procedure.

References

[1] *Points to Consider in the Production and Testing of New Drugs and Biologicals Produced by Recombinant DNA Technology.* Office of Biologics Research and Review, Center for Drugs and Biologics, Food and Drug Administration, 1985, and the supplement to the "Points to Consider in the Production and Testing of New Drugs and Biologicals Produced by Recombinant DNA Technology," April 6, 1992.

[2] *Points to Consider in the Characterization of Cell Lines Used to Produce Biologicals.* Office of Biologics Research and Review, Center for Drugs and Biologics, Food and Drug Administration, 1987.

[3] *Points to Consider in the Manufacture and Testing of Monoclonal Antibody Products for Human Use.* Office of Biologics Research and Review, Center for Drugs and Biologics, Food and Drug Administration, 1987.

[4]   *Cytokine and Growth Factor Pre-Pivotal Trial Information Package.* Center for Biologics Evaluation and Research, Food and Drug Administratin, April 1990.

[5]   *USP XXII /NF XXII.* Rockville, MD: The United States Pharmacopeial Convention, Inc., 1990.

[6]   Scopes, R.K. *Anal. Biochem. 59* (1974):277–282.

[7]   Whitaker, J.R. and Granum, P. E. *Anal. Biochem. 109* (1980):156–159.

[8]   *Notes to Applicants for Marketing Authorization on the Product and Quality Control of Medicinal Products Derived by Recombinant DNA Technology.* Committee for Proprietary Medicinal Products, March 1987.

[9]   Limulus Amebocyte Lysate Assay (PYOTELL) Product Package Insert, Associates of Cape Cod, Inc., Woods Hole, MA.

[10]   Title 21, Code of Federal Regulations, Sections 600–799. Washington, DC: Office of the Federal Register, National Archives and Records Administration, 1989.

7 Applied data analysis, sampling methodologies, and statistical validation techniques

G. R. Swartz

Contents

7.1 Introduction

The statistical way of thinking is actually an inverted approach to reality, where inductive versus deductive thinking is the rule. Theories are only useful when and if practical application is at hand. The more a theory claims global validity to reality, ironically the less applicable it becomes in verifying individual facts. The following quote may shed more light on this perspective:

> If, for instance, I determine the weight of each stone in a bed of pebbles and get an average weight of 145 grams, this tells me very little about the real nature of the pebbles. Anyone who thought, on the basis of these findings, that he could pick up a pebble of 145 grams at the first try would be in for a serious disappointment. Indeed, it might well happen that however long he searched, he would not find a single pebble weighing exactly 145 grams.
> —Dr. Carl Gustav Jung, 1958

The intent of this chapter is to provide the reader sound statistical principles with biotechnical examples. In this chapter, a person in the role of quality investigator will be able to see the use of empirical methods as they relate to real data.

7.2 Variation and error definitions

7.2.1 Variation defined

Things really do vary as they do. Variation is a fact in nature as well as in the work place. Think of the times you arrive at work or get up in the morning. Are you always exactly on time? The definition of variation is directly weighted by the factors that influence it.

Variation is fundamental to all sciences. In physics, variation is used to measure the dispersion of atomic particles. In agriculture, it is measured in the growth rates of produce yields and hybrids. The confidence in clinical studies is caused by and based upon variance. For example, assay variability can largely determine the outcome of a validation experiment. But, what are the types of variation that exist, and what causes things to vary so much? The reasons for variation can be broken down into two major categories., as shown in Table 7.1.

Table 7.1 Two major types of variation

Normal	Abnormal
Random	Nonrandom
Common causes	Special cases
Systematic	Localized
By Chance	Assignable cause
Expected	Irregular
Stable	Unstable
Unidentifiable	Identifiable

The USP XXII section on the "Design and Analysis of Biological Assays" [10] states that in minimizing the error variance in an assay, "test animals or their equivalent are then assigned at random but in equal numbers to different doses of the Standard and Unknown. This implies an objective random process, such as throwing dice, shuffling cards, or using a table of random numbers. Assigning the same number of individuals to each treatment simplifies the subsequent calculations materially, and usually leads to the shortest confidence interval for a given number of observations."

To observe variation, one must take into consideration an unbiased or random sample, an objective means of measuring, and a logical way of determining the causes of variation. Variation is the result of the output of a process. This result or dependent measurement is largely due to the variation in the components of the process.

Listed below are some of the process component sources of variation. They are similar to those found in cause and effect diagrams [1]:

1. people,
2. equipment,
3. materials,
4. methods,
5. environment, and
6. measurement.

7.2.2   Precision and accuracy defined

The terms "precision" and "accuracy" are sometimes construed to have the same meaning, but statistically they are very different. They represent two distinct attributes to gauge a process or parameter. *Precision* is defined as the degree of variation observed around a particular parameter, whereas *accuracy* is a function of how exactly on target a measurement is.

In the majority of cases, the degree of accuracy is affected to a large extent by calibration. "The intent of calibration is to rid or minimize bias in the measurement process"[2]. The degree of precision can be the same between a calibrated and an uncalibrated instrument, whereas the accuracy of an uncalibrated system will deliver erroneous results.

Biotechnical and chemical measurements are affected by these two components of precision and accuracy. In the diagram in Figure 7.1, the investigator can visualize the difference between these two important attributes in sampling a process or parameter.

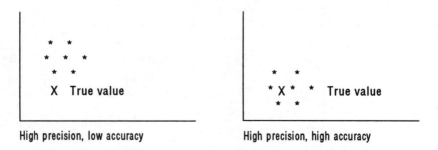

Figure 7.1 Differences between precision and accuracy

7.2.3   Types of errors

In discussing the various types of errors, two major categories of errors rise to the surface. They are systematic errors and random errors. In fact, these types of error correlate with the previous terms of accuracy and precision, respectively.

"Systematic errors are related to the particular measuring equipment involved" [3], whereas random errors exist by unpredictable and unknown variations in the process. Random errors are a source of noise in an experiment environment. Later in this chapter, an F test will be applied to assess the amounts of variance or randomness when comparing a control versus an experimental group.

The discussion of errors is especially relevant when comparing groups of biological test data versus a known population. The noise level, or amount of variance in an experimental situation, is directly related to its errors. Results from even the most sophisticated statistical analysis have little significance when error and noise are not accounted for or excluded altogether.

7.3   Estimating the standard deviation

7.3.1   Standard deviation, true variance

Variance and its effect on statistical results establishes the need for appropriate tools to estimate random variation for biotechnical applications. Given a normal distribution or bell shape population, it is possible to take a random sample of 30 or more units to estimate the variance of a process and/or product.

To demonstrate this, 30 temperature readings (T) were taken from three patients at ten-minute intervals after taking a drug. Sample data was calculated based upon the equation

$$X = 10 \ (T - 98 \ °F)$$

The calculated sample data (X) is as follows:

9	6	4	5	8	12	9	3	9	14	4	9	8	11	14	$N = 30$
5	5	9	7	3	4	5	8	9	12	14	8	9	11	14	

Determine the relative increase in temperature by adding the above readings and dividing the total by the sample size (N), which in this case is 30. An arithmetic mean equal to 8.267 is obtained. By dividing this average by 10, the time interval between readings, an average relative increase of 0.83 °F is realized after taking the drug.

The calculation of a standard deviation can be laborious; hence, it is recommended that a calculator or one of the many statistical software packages available be used to speed up this process. Descriptive statistics from a statistical software package such as Microstat® of the previous temperature readings are listed in Table 7.2 on the next page.

Not all of the information in the table is pertinent to this discussion, since the focus of this exercise is understanding variance, and not necessarily goodness of fit. The sample variance in Table 7.2 is calculated by dividing the deviation sum of squares (SS) by N - 1. When the square root of the sample variance is taken, the result is the sample standard deviation.

The standard deviation is an important statistic to garner, since it is the keystone for determining confidence intervals and creating statistical process control (SPC) chart guidelines.

Table 7.2 Descriptive statistics: temperature readings for patients after ingestion of drug

Variable name	=	Temp
N	=	30
Sample std. dev. (s)	=	3.41
Sample variance (s^2)	=	11.65
Coefficient of variation	=	41.28
Population std. dev.	=	3.35
Minimum	=	3
Maximum	=	14
Sum	=	248
Sum of squares	=	2388
Deviation SS	=	337.87

Normal distribution goodness of fit test:
The hypothesis that the population is normal of mean 8.27 and std. dev. 3.41 cannot be rejected at the 95% confidence level.

Chi square = 7.876, d.f. = 5, p = .1637

It is a general indicator of the amount of dispersion a process has. The larger the standard deviation, the greater the variance.

7.3.2 Coefficient of variation defined

The standard deviation depends on units as a measure of variation. However, in comparing the relative variation or whether the center weight of the distribution is influential on its variance, another tool called the coefficient of variation (*CV*) is recommended. The CV also is known as the unitless or dimensionless measure of variance.

$$CV = \frac{s}{\overline{X}}$$

Sometimes the *CV* is expressed as a percentage and the equation becomes:

$$\% \, CV = 100 \times \frac{s}{\overline{X}}$$

The coefficient can be used to compare changes in the same group of data or to compare the relative variability of two or more different sets of data. The group with the larger CV has the larger variability, as in the example below.

Group One: Standard deviation = 1.42 grams
             Average = 7.00 grams

Group Two: Standard deviation = 1.78 grams
                       Average = 10.00 grams

Question: Which group has the larger (relative) variability?

Upon initial inspection, it would appear that Group Two has more variance, but the center weight ,or average, has more relative impact on the variance. A *CV* study must be performed to correctly answer the question.

$$CV_1 = \frac{1.42}{7.00} = 0.203 \text{ or } 20.3\%$$

$$CV_2 = \frac{1.78}{10.00} = 0.178 \text{ or } 17.8\%$$

The conclusion is that, in fact, Group One has the larger relative variability. In retrospect, one must consider what question is really being asked before deciding whether to use the standard deviation or *CV* as an indicator for comparing variances. If the center weight has influence, then the *CV* would apply.

7.3.3   Central limit theorem and sampling distributions

In applying statistical tools to real data, an understanding of the Central Limit Theorem is recommended. This precept is best shown by example.

Figure 7.2 shows various distributions of dice thrown within the framework of a number of sample or group sizes, which hereinafter will be designated as n. In sample (a), for instance, one can see that the chance of finding any of the possible six outcomes are equally likely, so the sample has a nearly flat distribution.

The average $(\overline{X})$ of individual values tends to be normally distributed regardless of the individual (x) distribution. Another aspect is that the average of averages, or the grand average, is equivalent to the average of individuals when drawn from the same parent population—in this case, dice.

A sampling distribution is a distribution of averages. If randomly collected, the distribution will take on a nearly normal shape, which is advantageous when comparing a mean of an experimental group versus its control group or population. Another key element of this theory is the following equation:

Standard deviation of Averages× $\sqrt{n}$ = Standard deviation of Individuals   (1)

or

$$\sigma_{\overline{X}} \cdot \sqrt{n} = \sigma_x$$

Standard deviation of Individuals $+\sqrt{n}$ = Standard deviation of Averages   (2)

or

$$\sigma_{\overline{X}} = \frac{\sigma_x}{\sqrt{n}}$$

where n is the subgroup size or sample size.

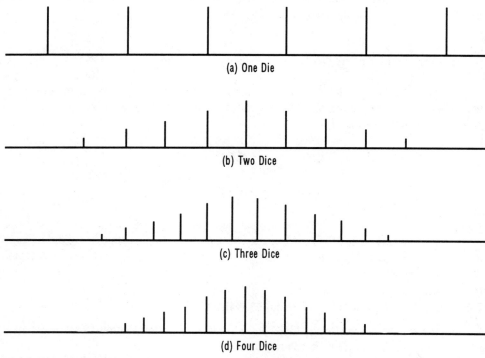

Figure 7.2 Various distributions of thrown dice

These equations become very useful in converting sampling distributions such as those from control charts to individual distributions. In this manner, one can convert and then compare individual distributions to the specification limits for yield determination and process capability studies.

Special Note: A pitfall exists in applying average distributions to specifications when, in fact, the investigator needs to apply the individual distribution for analysis with specification limits.

7.3.4 Confidence intervals for the standard deviation

When previous history of a process, or any distribution for that matter, is known, it may become desirable to establish a confidence interval for the variance of that process. The following is a cook book procedure to perform this interval. It is useful for establishing guidelines for chemical vendors or determining whether an experimental sample falls outside or inside an expected dispersion criteria.

In the example below and others to follow, statistical values from F, t, and Z statistical tables will be provided. To cross reference these values, please refer to "Tables for Statisticians" by Barnes & Nobel [11] for this chapter, or to the appropriate appendices at the end of the book.

Given: A process is normally distributed. A control sample size of 60 units has been drawn with a mean ($\overline{X}c$) of 13.5 and a standard deviation of 4.8. Based on the control sample results, it is possible to calculate a 90% confidence interval for the process standard deviation using the following procedure:

1a. From the F table (Appendix II), $F_{05} = 1.32$

1b. $F_{05} \leq \dfrac{\sigma_c^2}{\sigma^2}, \ \sigma \leq \sqrt{\dfrac{\sigma_c^2}{F_{05}}} \ , \ \sigma \leq \sqrt{\dfrac{(4.8)^2}{1.32}}$

1c. Substituting, $\sigma \leq 4.178$

Note: The tabled values of both F_{05} and F_{95} are used to determine the 90% confidence level. Typically most tables for F values are greater than 1, therefore F_{05} can be pulled directly from Appendix II. It is selected by using the appropriate degrees of freedom, e.g., 59 and ∞. To determine F_{95}, the reciprocal value of F_{05} is used as follows.

2a. From the F table, $F_{95} = \dfrac{1}{1.32} = .757$

2b. $F_{95} \geq \dfrac{\sigma_c^2}{\sigma^2}, \ \sigma \geq \sqrt{\dfrac{\sigma_c^2}{F_{95}}}$

2c. Substituting, $\sigma \geq 5.517$

3. $4.178 \leq \sigma \leq 5.517$ with 90% Confidence. Hence, one would be relatively certain (90%) that the standard deviation would be within the stated range of 4.178 to 5.517.

7.3.5 Confidence intervals for the mean

Since sampling distributions have a central tendency, the user can establish confidence intervals around the grand average. Refer to Appendix I to obtain the appropriate Z score (standard deviate) to establish say a 95% confidence interval ($\alpha = .05$) around some critical parameter of interest. The corresponding Z value you find should be 1.96.

   Confidence intervals for the mean are set up in manner very similar to that discussed for the variance or standard deviation. The confidence interval for both small and large sample means can be established.

7.3.5.1 Sample sizes greater than 30

1. Determine the appropriate Z value for 95 or 99% confidence ($\alpha = .05$ or $.01$).

2.   Determine the sampling error: $\pm Z \left(\dfrac{s}{\sqrt{n}} \right)$

   where s is the sample standard deviation.

3.   Determine confidence interval: $\overline{X} - Z \left(\dfrac{s}{\sqrt{n}} \right) < \overline{X} < \overline{X} + Z \left(\dfrac{s}{\sqrt{n}} \right)$

   A process change has been implemented to improve the extrusion characteristics of a viscous solution from a syringe. Given the following summary statistical data, provide a realistic picture of what could be expected of future mean extrusion data with 95% confidence.

Summary Data: Interval $= \overline{X} - Z \left(\frac{s}{\sqrt{n}}\right) < \overline{X} < \overline{X} + Z \left(\frac{s}{\sqrt{n}}\right)$

$\overline{X} = 18 \, kgf$
$s = 4 \, kgf.$
$n = 103$

$Z_{95} = 1.96$ Substituting, $17.228 < \overline{X} < 18.773$

Hence, one could say that 95% of the time, or 19 out of 20 lots, one would expect to see mean extrusion between 17.228 and 18.773 kgf.

Besides the normal Z distribution there is another important probability function called the Student's t distribution or, simply, the t distribution). This distribution was first introduced by W.S. Gosset in 1908 when working for a brewery in England. Like the Z distribution, the t distribution is bell-shaped with its mean, medium, and mode coinciding at 0, but the t distribution is more dispersed as a function of the sample size pulled and, thus, the degrees of freedom $(n - 1)$ are affected. While there is only one standard normal distribution, there are a whole family of t distributions.

The investigator can use this distribution to great advantage, especially when the sample size is an economic consideration. Figure 7.3 shows the effect of sample size.

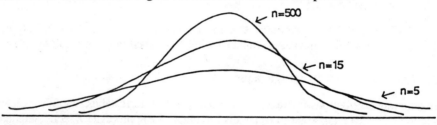

Figure 7.3 Effect of sample size on the student's t distribution

7.3.5.2 Sample sizes less than 30

1. Determine the appropriate t value for 95 or 99% confidence ($\alpha = .05$ or $.01$).

2. Determine the sampling error: $\pm t \left(\frac{s}{\sqrt{n}}\right)$

3. Determine the confidence interval: $\overline{X} - t \left(\frac{s}{\sqrt{n}}\right) < \overline{X} < \overline{X} + t \left(\frac{s}{\sqrt{n}}\right)$

Summary Data:

$\overline{X} = 8.45 \, lb$
$s = 1.32 \, lb$
$n = 15$

$t_{95} = 2.145$ Substituting, $7.72 < \overline{X} < 9.18$

Note: Degrees of freedom (df) $= n-1$, so the tabled t_{95} value is found at df $= 14$ and $\alpha = 0.05$.

Hence, one could say that 95% of time, or 19 out of 20 lots, one would expect to see means between 7.72 and 9.18 lb, with a sample size $n = 15$.

7.4   Cookbook comparison techniques

In relating comparative techniques to the previous section on confidence intervals, this section presents hypothesis testing as an approach to the initial design of experiments. This section presents a structure for both mean and variance comparisons. For further reading, please refer to the reference section [4].

7.4.1   Hypothesis testing

The test of hypothesis can be utilized in the following applications:
1. Variance comparison: F test
2. Mean comparison: t and Z test
3. Analysis of variance (ANOVA)
   a.   One-way ANOVA
   b.   Two-way ANOVA

   Hypothesis testing is really the cornerstone of statistical inference. In simple experiments, the hypothesis is stated about differences between mean values and also differences in the variation.
1. Establish the null and alternative hypothesis:
   Null Hypothesis = H_0 Alternative Hypothesis = H_1
2. Specify the test statistic.
3. Select the level of significance (α) for the test and the size (n).
4. State the decision rule for the test.
5. Draw a random sample of size n from the population.
6. Compute the value of the test statistic from the sample.
7. Accept or reject H_0 according to the decision rule.

7.4.2   Variance comparison

A procedure often missed in the comparison of two sets of data or two groups is the F test. This method provides the investigator with a step-by-step approach for comparing two groups of data. Below is a cookbook method for variance comparisons and the procedure for performing the F test.

7.4.2.1   Example of variance comparison using F test

A manager asks an investigator to check out a new supplier for HCl because of lower cost. The investigator is satisfied with the present supplier since they typically ship material with little pH variability from lot to lot. The investigator must determine whether the variability of the new supplier is significantly different than that of the present supplier with 95% confidence. A technician provides the investigator with pH data from the current supplier's past ten samples, which were found to have pH variance of $0.87\ S^2_{current}$, while the new supplier has a variance of $0.30\ S^2_{new}$ in a sample size of 15. Note: The variance is the square of the standard deviation.

1. Calculate the F value, $F = \dfrac{S^2_c}{S^2_n} = \dfrac{0.87}{0.30} = 2.9$

2. Pulling the F value from the table, at $\alpha = 0.05$, $F = 2.65$
3. Since the calculated F value of 2.9 exceeds the tabled value of 2.65, there is a significant difference in the variances of the two suppliers.
4. The new supplier has a significantly narrower variance.

In this example, the new supplier's variance is significantly better (lower); however, it may be recommended that the test be replicated, if economically feasible, to validate the results.

7.4.3 Mean comparison

The F test is normally performed to initially determine the difference in the spread or dispersion of two or more groups of data. Sequentially, mean comparison studies help the investigator discover differences in the aim or central tendency between groups of data.

Suppose an investigator has two groups of yield data containing equal sample sizes, as in the example summarized below. Upon performing the F test, no significant difference is found in the variances as $F = 1.24$. Performing a pooled t test with a pooled standard deviation helps determine whether Group Two has a significant yield improvement.

7.4.3.1 Example of mean comparison using t test with a pooled standard deviation

Summary Data:

	Group One	Group Two
Mean	77.14	88.21
Standard deviation	1.50	1.87
Sample (n)	10	10

1. Calculate mean difference: $88.21 - 77.14 = 11.07$
2. Calculate pooled standard deviation (S_p):

$$S_p = \sqrt{\frac{(n_1 - 1)\,\sigma_1^2 + (n_2 - 1)\,\sigma_2^2}{n_1 + n_2 - 2}} = 1.695$$

3. Solve for t: $\dfrac{\overline{X_1} - \overline{X_2}}{S_p \sqrt{\dfrac{1}{n_1} - \dfrac{1}{n_2}}} = 14.60$

4. Determine d.f. for pooled data: $(n_1 + n_2 - 2) = 18$

   where $\sqrt{\dfrac{1}{n_1} - \dfrac{1}{n_2}}$ is the correction factor.

5. Compare calculated t value with tabled value of 2.878 at 99% confidence.

Since the difference in the variances is not significant, the investigator has pooled the standard deviation. The t value of 14.6 is large; hence, it can be concluded that the yield of Group Two is significantly improved over Group One with 99% confidence. This type of test can be used in comparing yields, differences in chemical solutions, or to determine the significance of treatment conditions.

> Any theory based on experience is necessarily statistical; that is to say, it formulates an ideal average which abolishes all exceptions at either end of the scale and replaces them by an abstract mean. This mean is quite valid, though it need not necessarily occur in reality.
>
> —C.G. Jung, 1958

The above quote may shed some light on the way we determine significant results. If the mean is valid, replication may indeed still be recommended to further validate findings and solidify results.

7.4.4 Summary guidelines for comparison studies and confidence intervals

The following outline provides a summary of concepts on both confidence intervals and comparison studies presented in this chapter.

Confidence intervals
1. Intervals around $\bar{X}$
2. Generation of interval around 0
3. Intervals around variable and attribute data

Variance comparison
1. Detects changes in spread of process
2. Utilizes F ratio
3. Provides theoretical basis for ANOVA

Mean comparison studies
1. Detects shifts in aim of process
2. Utilizes Z and t statistics
   Z test when sample $n > 30$
   t test when sample $n < 30$
3. Similarity to confidence intervals

Examples include:
   Analysis of chemical data, pH values, temperature, etc.
   Using mean comparison in yield data
   Estimating population defect density, particulate levels

7.5 Process capability—yield enhancement

7.5.1 Comparing specifications to data

In applying process capability for biotechnical industries, firms often examine the constraints and terms of some FDA requirement. For example, the USP Section on "Experimental Error and Tests of Assay Validity" [10] discusses error variance of an individual response as follows:

> In the Pharmacopeial assays, differences in dose that modify the mean response are assumed not to affect the variability in the response. The calculation of the error variance depends upon the design of the assay and the form of the adjustment for any missing values. Each response is first converted to the unit Y used in computing the potency. Determine a single error variance from the combined deviations of the t's around their respective means for each dosage level, summed over all levels.

The discussion of error variance in the USP is pertinent here in terms of how large the relative variance is and the way it is calculated. In many cases, this determines the outcome of the process capability study. According to the USP, "doubtful values of Y may be tested as described under 'Rejection of Outlying or Aberrant Observations', and proved outliers may be replaced as 'Missing Values'."

Relating this to applied data analysis and the validation of results, yield and process capability studies become effective in the determination of accept/reject criteria. As an added value, the results may actually help in meeting or exceeding the criteria for pharmaceutical or medical devices.

The discussion earlier on variation relates in terms of comparing a distribution with its specifications. On a unit-by-unit (individual) basis, one needs to consider the individual

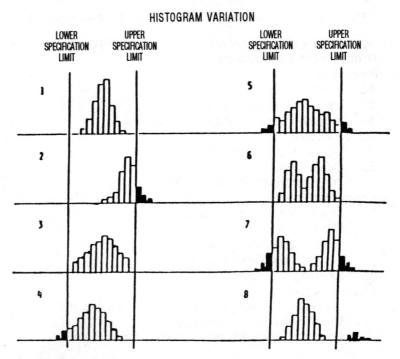

Figure 7.4 Comparisons of distributions with their respective specifications

distribution when performing the analysis. If, for example, one looks at the following distributions (Figure 7.4) and compares them to their respective specification limits, which situation appears to be most desirable?

The first one (1) is correct, because even if the process shifted a little in either direction, there would still be enough tolerance. It is recommended that the distribution of data be visually inspected prior to performing a yield enhancement study.

7.5.2   Yield enhancement and process capability

Ideally, if only normal distributions existed, one might not be overly concerned with process variation. But, because of outliers or non-normal distributions, it is recommended that the steps outlined below be implemented for a yield enhancement study:

1. Take a minimum of 30 samples up front and run a goodness of fit test such as a Chi square test for normalcy or a probability plot.
2. Perform process capability or yield determination study.
3. Take corrective action on outliers or obvious anomalies in the data.
4. Perform process capability study once more to determine improved yield.

7.5.2.1 Yield determination using Z or t statistics

When the total sample $n \leq 30$, a recommended procedure is to use the student's t distribution. Using the procedure below, the current yield on a product or process parameter can be determined.

Summary Statistics:

Mean of product's weight	5 lb
Product's standard deviation	.50 lb
Total sample size n	10
Upper spec.	5.75 lb
Lower spec.	4.25 lb

1. Determine df: $n - 1 = 9$
2. Determine t of upper spec. (US): $\dfrac{US - \overline{X}}{S} = \dfrac{5.75 - 5}{.5} = 1.5$

3. Determine t of Lower Spec. (LS): $\dfrac{\overline{X} - LS}{S} = \dfrac{5 - 4.25}{.5} = 1.5$

4. From t table, derive (α) area that falls outside specification limits. Since area of 8.4% is beyond each specification, multiply by 2. This is the reject area, or 16.8% rejectable. The area beyond lower and upper specifications = 0.084 x 2 = 0.168

5. Yield = (1 − Area in Step 4) = 0.832 or 83.2%

7.5.3 Process capability

Different statisticians, companies, and QC texts use varying formulas to determine process capability indices. However, all have a common thread in that the formulas are based upon conventional statistical theory and probability distributions.

Basic capability (C_p) and process capability (C_{pk}) indices show how well a process is meeting its specification guidelines. They generally point to the fact that 99.73% of the output of a critical parameter will fall within plus or minus three standard deviations of the mean of that parameter. The common base for computing the C_p is the six standard deviations width.

Process capability indices provide a simple yet effective method for determining how well a biotechnical product performs to its specifications, as shows in the example below.

7.5.3.1 Example of process capability determination

Hardness of water is measured in terms of the amount of calcium ion concentration (in parts per million). Given the following hypothetical hardness specifications, determine if the water can meet this specification 99.73% of the time.

Summary Statistics:		Specifications:	
Average	136.4	Upper Spec.	140.0
Standard deviation	1.2	Lower Spec.	130.0

Use Cp index: $C_p = \dfrac{US - LS}{6\sigma} = \dfrac{10}{7.2} = 1.38$

Calculate the C_{pk} index if process is not precisely centered within specification tolerance (e.g., 135 ppm). C_{pk} is equal to the minimum of the following:

$$\frac{US - \overline{X}}{3\sigma} = \frac{3.6}{3.6} = 1.0$$

or

$$\frac{\overline{X} - LS}{3\sigma} = \frac{6.4}{3.6} = 1.78$$

The process capability index, C_{pk}, is equal to 1.0, meaning that the minimum upper spec index still falls exactly on three standard deviations of the distribution of calcium ion concentration. Therefore, the water can meet this hardness specification 99.73% of the time. The latter percentage can also be considered the yield of this hard water.

7.6 Sampling methods and applications

CFR 211.84 (b)(6) discusses the sampling required to test component, drug product containers, and closures as follows:

> "Representative samples of each shipment of each lot shall be collected for testing or examination. The number of containers to be sampled, and the amount of material to be taken from each container, shall be based upon appropriate criteria such as statistical criteria for component variability, confidence levels and degree of precision desired, the past quality history of the supplier, and the quantity needed for analysis...."

For final product testing that is destructive to the product, some statistical sample methods are not appropriate if too many units are destroyed in order to reach the desired confidence level. A final product sterility test on an aseptically filled product is such an example. In this case, samples should be pulled from the first, middle and last parts of the fill. This type of sampling represents cross sections of the batch and is also useful in testing for content uniformity.

7.6.1 Quality levels and errors

The following terms and definitions may help clarify the plethora of various quality terms surrounding sampling plans, their statistical errors, and confidence levels.

ACCEPTABLE QUALITY LEVEL (AQL):   The term refers to a 95% confidence in a specific fraction defective of interest. The alpha error of this plan is always 5% unless otherwise specified. This level is especially affected by the acceptance criteria. For example, the less rejects acceptable in a sampling plan, the lower the fraction defective. The 5% risk is in rejecting material which is truly acceptable and is considered to be the producer's risk. The AQL was developed through Mil-Std-105D.

LOT TOLERANCE PERCENT DEFECTIVE (LTPD):   The 90% confidence level in rejecting a product that is truly bad. The 10% error is always 10% unless otherwise extrapolated. Truly this LTPD level is quite often misunderstood, for the concept is reversed in that the consumer will be confident nine out of ten times that a product appearing to be of poor quality really is an undesirable fraction defective. The 10% risk lies in accepting material of poor quality and is often referred to as the consumer's risk. The LTPD was conceived via Mil-Std 38510 in conjunction with the Poisson distribution.

AVERAGE OUTGOING QUALITY LEVEL (AOQL):   This level is experienced after sampling has taken place. Generally, the AOQL is based upon the fraction defective coming into the plan and its relative probability of acceptance.

INDIFFERENCE QUALITY LEVEL (IQL):   This level is at the 50% probability of acceptance on an operating characteristic (OC) curve and is associated with the AOL. This in all practicality is the worse or weakest point on an OC Curve.

7.6.2 Sampling plans applicable to biotechnology

It is fairly costly to attempt to sample quality into a product. Not only are sampling plans misunderstood, they are also in some cases applied to processes that are totally out of statistical control. In fact, wherever possible, it is recommended to implement SPCs [5].

The application of sampling plans to biotechnology actually are quite numerous and, when applied, should be implemented with rigor. A suggested reference, especially when the fractions of interest exceed below 10%, is the LTPD plans based upon the Poisson distribution. As an added plus, the associated AQL is provided in parentheses (See Mil-Std 38510H for details).

7.6.2.1 Sampling plan example

Recently, a biotechnical firm desired to guarantee with 95% confidence that their solutions in vials contained no more than 700 ppm of zinc. For inspection of the samples, an atomic absorption spectrophotometer was employed. What sample size is appropriate to detect this 700 ppm level? [Hint: 700 ppm = 0.07%]

From an LTPD table, using an acceptance number (c) = 0 and the associated AQL in parentheses of 0.07%, the required sample size is 76, or 76 vials.

Subsequently, the firm discovered a new spectrophotometer that can perform multiple samples at a faster rate and that the sample size could be increased to 153. Using the same table, we can determine with 95% confidence the sensitivity of detection. In other words, what ppm level of zinc could be detectable?

Again, from a Poisson table, using an acceptance number (c) = 0 and finding a sample as large as 153, it is determined that the associated AQL is at 0.03% or 300 ppm, with this sampling plan in mind.

7.6.2.2 Summary sampling thoughts

Although the investigator needs to be alerted to instances where SPC can be applied, sampling plans and methods may become a necessity to meet FDA requirements of a product's outgoing quality. Some things to keep in mind when applying sampling plans are listed below:

1. Never believe that quality can be sampled into a product. Quality is something that is built into a product.
2. The use of a sampling plan is needed to find an appropriate sample size or detection level, an empirical plan such as the Poisson plan presented in this chapter should be used.
3. When working with vendors and/or customers, always investigate possibilities for statistical analysis of data versus attribute sampling schemes.

7.7 Validation of analytical methods

It is the purpose of this section to address the statistical treatment of *variability* of analytical methods. Other method validation issues, such as specificity, limit of detection, limit of quantitation, linearity, interference, and enhancement of specific biotechnical assays, will not be addressed.

7.7.1 Goal of validation techniques

The goal of a manufacturer of biotechnology products is reproducibility within acceptable specified limits. CFR 211.160 (b)(6) says:

> Laboratory controls shall include the establishment of sound and appropriate specification, standards, sampling plans, and test procedures designed to assure that components, drug product containers, closures, in-process materials, labeling and drug products conform to appropriate standards of identity, strength, quality and purity....

CFR 211.165 (e) continues by stating that "the accuracy, sensitivity, and reproducibility of test methods employed by the firm shall be established and documented."

7.7.2 Variability of analytical methods

Analytical methods can be inherently variable. Test results can vary from analyst to analyst, from instrument to instrument, or from day to day. Yet, these are the same test results that are used to check critical steps in the manufacturing process and to determine if the final product meets specifications and can be used in humans. A properly designed validation experiment can help identify the causes and extent of assay variability. The analyst must then determine if the variability is acceptable or not and decide what steps to take to improve reproducibility of results.

As an example, suppose the specification for an active ingredient is ±10% of the amount claimed on the product label. The validation of an analytical assay gave a total variability of ±10% for the test method.

The experimenter may ask the following question: How would one know if a passing result was actually within the specification or if a failing result was outside of the specification? Either result could be an artifact of the variability inherent in the assay, and one could accept bad material or fail good material. It is important that the total variability on any analytical procedure be significantly less than the specification range.

7.7.3 Experimental error and tests of assay validity

In reference to the inclusion of experimental error, USP states:

> As the term is used here, "experimental error" refers to the residual variation in the response of biological indicators, not to a mistake in procedure or to an outlier that needs replacement. It is measured in terms of the error variance of a single response or other unit, which is designated uniformly as S Squared, despite differences in the definition of the unit. It is required in tests of assay validity and in computing the confidence interval.

A good analytical procedure is consistently reproducible when performed by trained individuals using properly calibrated instrumentation. Those products regulated by the Center for Biological Research must be tested and certified by the FDA before they can be released for sale—another reason for methods to be properly validated for reproducibility. Such validation will provide confidence that the FDA can duplicate an experiment's results using the experimentor's own procedures.

The example in the next section illustrates an analytical method validation of an assay using gas chromatography. There were two analysts trained to perform this test with only one chromatograph. The investigator wants to know if there is a significant difference from one analyst to the other, or from the same analyst performing the test on different days.

Except for the variable being tested, all other variables must be held constant. For example, all tests for the validation must be performed on material from the same manufactured lot of product, eliminating lot-to-lot variability. The intent here is to minimize both extrinsic and intrinsic forms of variability that could bias results from the experiment.

The purpose of the following example is to show how assay variability is affected by measurement mediums such as gas chromatography (GC) or high-pressure liquid chromatography (HPLC). For demonstration purposes, let us use GC to measure concentration strength of cortisone acetate in the example.

7.7.4 Data and variance analysis

Analysis of variance (ANOVA) is employed as a method to determine if day-to-day variances of instrumentation or procedures and their analysts have any significant effect on the outcome of the HPLC assays. The two main factors under consideration are (1) day-to-day variances, and (2) person-to-person variances.

The purpose of this hypothetical study is two-fold. Firstly, it will determine if the factors of days and persons are significant; secondly, the study will determine if the overall assay variability of HPLC in this instance exceeds the specification requirements.

In this example case, cortisone acetate must be within a specified label tolerance between 97 and 102%, with an average concentration strength of 3.0 mg/ml. All data are listed in mg of cortisone acetate per ml of sample.

Hypothesis Statements:
1. Variances between the two analysts are not significant.
2. Variances from one day to another are not significant.

Data Analysis:

	Ingrid	**Dirk**	**Totals**
Day 1	3.24	3.19	
	3.27	3.15	
	<u>3.25</u>	<u>3.16</u>	
Sum	**9.76**	**9.50**	**19.26**
Average	3.25	3.17	
Std. dev.	0.02	0.02	
Day 2	3.15	3.35	
	2.95	3.16	
	<u>3.13</u>	<u>3.18</u>	
Sum	**9.23**	**9.69**	**18.92**
Average	3.08	3.23	
Std. dev.	0.10	0.10	
Totals	**18.99**	**19.19**	**38.18**

Without laboring through sum of squares calculations at this point, the ANOVA table presents the results (see Table 7.3).

Table 7.3 ANOVA results

Source	SS	df	MS	F
Day	0.010	1	0.010	2.50
Person	0.003	1	0.003	0.75
Day x Person	0.056	1	0.056	14.00
Error	0.035	8	0.004	
TOTAL	0.104			

$F_{1,8}$ (a= .05) = 5.32 (tabled F value)

MS = mean square = $\dfrac{SS}{df}$

7.7.5 Analysis of HPLC experimental results

The ANOVA revealed to the investigator the following results:
1. Since day-to-day F value did not exceed the tabled value (2.5 < 5.32), day-to-day variance is not significant.
2. Since person-to-person F value did not exceed the tabled value (.75 < 5.32), person-to-person variance is not significant.
3. However, the interaction F value (day x person) exceeded the tabled value (14.0 > 5.32), indicating that the interaction variance of these two factors is significant.

The investigator can conclude from this HPLC study that the two isolated factors of interest, persons and days, have no significant effect on the outcome of the assay. However, what is interesting is the interaction between the factors. Therefore, it is recommended that this experiment be replicated again with a different analyst performing the assay to see if replication of results is perceived.

Besides the interaction finding, also of particular significance is the overall degree of precision of the assay results. By determining this precision and the total assay variance, one can decide if the material in question, cortisone acetate, is within the specification tolerance.

The largest standard deviation of 0.1 mg/ml is used from a single triplicate run. The precision of the assay is defined by:

Average ±0.1 (mg/ml cortisone acetate) = 3.2 ±0.1

The total assay variance is defined as:

±(grand mean - expected mean) ±precision

or   [± (3.2 – 3.0) ±0.1] mg/ml = ±0.3 mg/ml

Taking this analysis one step further, the investigator can look back at the original specification and compare it to the results. Inherently, one can readily perceive a shift in the assay mean versus the expected mean, (e.g., 3.2 versus 3.0).

The specification width of 97 to 102 % runs from 2.91 to 3.06 around the expected mean of 3.0. The conclusion is that both assay variance and the compound itself (X = 3.2) fall outside the specification tolerance. Hence, the results of this particular experiment invalidated both the assay and the compound.

7.8 Summary concepts in experimental design

In the last example for establishing the variability associated with HPLC, a simple two-way ANOVA was employed. This brief section is a cursory overview of some of the terms and definitions associated with factorial and experimental design. For more detail into empirical approaches, and design considerations, a suggested reference is Box, Hunter, and Hunter's *Statistics for Experimenters* [7].

7.8.1 Factorial design terms and definitions

RESPONSE (DEPENDENT) VARIABLE: The variable to be studied and optimized.

FACTOR (INDEPENDENT) VARIABLE: A variable that may affect the values of the response variable.

LEVEL (TREATMENT):   A certain numerical value of a factor.

REPLICATES: Multiple measurements of the response variable for each combination of different levels of factors.

STATISTICAL DESIGN OF EXPERIMENTS (SDE):   For given response variables, Factors, and levels of each factor, measurements of response variable(s) are taken for all or some combination of different levels of factors to determine:
1. Whether a factor or an interaction of factors has a significant (at some prefixed significance level) effect on the response variable(s), and
2. How a significant factor/interaction is impacting the response variable(s), and
3. Optimal levels of factors for best results of response variables.
   a.   The statistical tool used for 1 is ANOVA.
   b.   Normal equations to determine the response surface are used for 2 and 3.

7.8.2 2^2 factorial designs

For a response variable to be studied, two independent variables or factors are chosen. Each factor takes two different levels (settings). Thus, there are four different combinations of levels of factors, and for each combination, measurement(s) of the response variable is (are) taken. The previous validation assay serves as an example of this design. The objective is to determine whether each factor or the interaction has a significant effect on the response variable in the experiment.

7.8.3 Summary of basic experimental methods

This section reviews of some of the basic experimental design principles and statistical methods with application to the biotechnical environment. The following list is a brief summary of these comparative techniques for significance testing:
1. Covariance testing,
2. Mean Comparative Test,
3. Variance Comparison Studies, and
4. Analysis of Variance
   a.   One-way—used with more than two groups of data.
   b.   Two-way—allows for interaction effects and provides basis for factorial designs.

7.9   Statistical process control primer and reference tool

This guide addresses the seemingly complex ideas and concepts of SPC in a format which is perhaps easier to understand than previously presented. The purpose is to define SPC principles in a fashion that is readily perceived and easy to comprehend.

7.9.1   What is SPC?

What is SPC, and why is the title written "statistical process control" instead of "statistical quality control" (SQC)? Briefly, SQC's other name is SPC, or statistical process control. In other words, SQC's main function is process control. With the aid of control charts, one can learn to control a process, improve yields, reduce waste, and, in the final analysis, save money.

7.9.2   Introduction to terms and definitions

Ahead lie some of the basic words/terminology to prime the potential investigator before venturing off on a journey to process control. The list includes SPC terms that may have specific application in a biotechnical environment.

ACCEPTANCE CRITERIA: Refers generally to the amount of acceptable rejects before a lot will be rejected based on the sample that is drawn. Used in sampling plans as the criteria for passing or failing a lot of items inferred from the sample.

ACCEPTABLE QUALITY LEVEL (AQL):   Refers to a coordinate point for the fraction defective on the x axis of the operating characteristic curve of an attribute sampling plan. This point is the region of good quality and reasonably low rejection probability—5% alpha error— therefore, a 95% probability of acceptance.

ACCURACY: Webster defines accuracy and precision as one and the same, when in fact, they are not. Accuracy is how close a measurement comes to its actual value. In a particular process, accuracy could be a function of calibration . See Precision.

ALPHA ERROR: The probability of error in making an assumption incorrectly. In sampling plans, it is the probability of rejecting a lot which is truly good. In hypotheses testing, it refers to the mistake we make by rejecting the null hypothesis when, in fact, it is true. In control charts, it is the assumption that a process point is out-of-control, when it is not, and is due to statistical chance alone. Therefore, the smaller the alpha error in any case, the more confidence we have in the result(s) obtained.

ANALYSIS: Implies some conclusion based on statistical results in order to interpret some meaning from the statistical test (s) performed; interpretation.

AMBIENT: Refers to certain intervening variables in an environment that have some effect on the result being measured. Generally, ambient variables or factors in an industrial environment are those which are not wanted in any particular experiment. Examples of ambient variables could be dust particles, ambient temperatures, or ambient sources of light.

ARITHMETIC AVERAGE: Also known as the mean of the distribution, it is a measure of central tendency indicating the center weight of a distribution of scores. Think of a scale which is always level, regardless of the distribution of scores along a line, and holding that scale up so that it is always balanced. This is the weighting factor or center of any distribution of scores.

ASSIGNABLE CAUSES: Those causes of problems that are sporadic in nature and not due to statistical chance alone. Assignable causes are ones which can be assigned a reason as to why that problem point exists. Usually, points outside of control chart limits are those associated with some assignable cause, this cause being of a sporadic nature and identifiable.

ATTRIBUTE DATA: Qualitative data based on the absence or presence of some characteristic, usually determined by some specification. Common types of attribute data would include: go/no-go data, pass-fail, accept-reject, yield-reject, etc. Attribute data is based on a binomial population of mutually exclusive events designated by P and $Q = 1 - P$.

AVERAGE OUTGOING QUALITY (AOQ):   Based upon the fraction defective (P) and the probability of acceptance (PA) for that fraction defective, also taking into the account the characteristics of an attribute sampling plan, that is, its sample size and decision criteria. $AOQ = P(A) \times P$.

AVERAGE OUTGOING QUALITY LIMIT (AOQL):   The threshold point on the AOQ curve. It is the worst possible case outgoing quality and is generally derived from the area of indifference of the operating characteristic curve.

BETA ERROR: In sampling plans, beta error is associated with the LTPD point and implies a 10% risk in accepting a lot that is truly rejectable. In hypothesis testing, it is the error made in rejecting an alternative hypothesis when in fact, it is true. In control charts, beta is the error made in assuming the process is in control when, in fact, it is not.

BIMODAL DISTRIBUTION: A distribution having two modes depicted by two distinctive humps in the curve. The presence of two frequently occurring scores, or groups of scores, is noticeable.

BINOMIAL DISTRIBUTION: A discrete probability distribution for attribute data that applies to the conformance and noncomformance of units. This distribution also is the basis for attribute control charts such as p and np charts.

CAPABILITY: Refers to the process capability study of whether or not product is truly capable of conforming to specifications. This capability can be determined only after the process is in statistical control. A process may be defined as being truly capable when the aim of the process is well centered and the variance or spread of the process on an individual unit basis does not exceed the specification limits.

CAUSE AND EFFECT DIAGRAM: A simple tool for individual or group problem-solving that uses a graphic description of the various process elements to analyze potential sources of process variation; also called a fishbone diagram (because of its appearance) developed by Ishikawa.

CAPRICIOUS DATA: The naturally occurring chaos in all things, or the unexpected results one derives from attempting to sort out dirty data. Capricious means sudden shifts, or abnormal changes.

CENTRAL LIMIT THEOREM (CLT):   States that when collecting a distribution of averages or subgroup scores, the distribution will tend to centralize around the center value. In other words, the distribution will be evenly distributed about the mean or average. This is true even if the averages are sampled from an abnormal distribution (skewed, bimodal, etc.).

CONTROL: To take command of a situation is the dictionary definition; however, in reference to SQC, control means to get a handle on the process and be able to manipulate it in a desirable fashion.

CONTROL CHARTS: A tool in which one can visualize a particular process over time and/or across units. It is a way to graphically represent a parameter in an unbiased manner. The various types of control charts are as follows:

C CHARTS: Used to depict the number of defects per *unit*. For example, the number of defects per automobile. An average number of defects per automobile can also be obtained ($\overline{C}$).

P CHARTS: Used when the percent or fraction defective is graphically desired. It depicts the fraction defection per sample, and an average can be obtained.

NP CHARTS: Used to depict the number of defects per sample. Similar to a C chart, NP easily counts the number of defects, which makes charting fairly simple. The main requirement for a NP chart is that the sample size must remain constant.

R CHARTS: Used to monitor the range variation when collecting averaged or subgroup data. Usually seen in conjunction with an X bar chart, the range chart gives information to the variance of a process over time, across units, or across samples.

S CHARTS: Similar to R charts and measure the process variation via the sample standard deviations. The S chart is especially applicable with larger sample sizes.

X BAR CHARTS: Are used to monitor variables data (continuous variables) over time. Generally, X Bar Charts, graphically represent averages or groups of data over time. They serve as a good indication of any particular process which has been identified either as a problem area, or for monitoring purposes.

CONTROL LIMITS: The boundary lines set up on any control chart for the purpose of determining whether or not a process is in or out of control Typically, the area between the control limits account for 99.7% of the distribution of scores making up the control chart. When control limits are set plus and minus three sigma (standard deviations), it will accommodate again 99.7% of the distribution.

CONTROL LIMITS FOR AVERAGES: Used for averages on an X chart, when taking average or subgroup data. They also serve as a boundary parameter for a majority of the scores being marked down on the chart (99.7%), but in this case it applies for averages and not individual scores.

CONTROL LIMITS FOR INDIVIDUALS: Also known as the natural process limits, they help determine, again with 99.7% confidence, where the expected process will go. Because these limits are for individual scores, they will assist in determining the yield for a particular process.

FAULT-TREE ANALYSIS: A brainstorming and communication tool to figure out all the possible causes of any particular yield, productivity, or quality problem. This tool uses a fishbone diagram to analyze all of the possible causes to an identified problem in the categorized areas of people, equipment, specifications, flow, raw materials, and measurement.

KURTOSIS: Refers to the height of a distribution of scores. Platykurtic means a flat and very dispersed distribution, whereas leptokurtic means a tall and very tightened distribution.

LOT TOLERANCE PERCENT DEFECTIVE (LTPD):   This particular defective level is guaranteed with 90% confidence of meeting the plan, and a 10% beta error or probability of rejection. See beta error.

MEAN: Same as arithmetic average.

MEASURE: Dictionary defines measure as the dimensions, quantity, or capacity of anything ascertained by a scale or by the variable condition. In SPC, measure could be a reference standard or a sample used for the quantitative comparison of properties.

MEDIAN: The middle score when the scores are ranked from highest to lowest or lowest to highest. When the median is resolved half of the scores will be on one side and the other half on the other side.

METHODOLOGY: The systematic way in which an application is addressed to a problem. SPC methodology involves a logical approach with statistical tools to effectively solve problems.

MIDPOINT: In reference to cell intervals, it is the middle point of any particular cell.

MODIFIED CONTROL LIMITS: Generally performed when the process is well within the specification limits and both the upper and lower specification limits are outside the natural limits of the process.

MODE: A measure of central tendency indicating where the most frequently occurring score or group of scores lies in a distribution.

NORMAL: A continuous, symmetrical, bell-shaped frequency distribution for variables data which is the basis for control charts for variables. The mean, median, and mode are approximately the same, and a standard deviation (S) exists where plus and minus one $S = 68\%$, plus and minus two $S = 95\%$, and plus and minus three $S = 99.7\%$, which is a standard setting for control charts limits.

PARETO CHART: A simple tool for problem-solving that involves making all potential problem areas or sources of variation. Pareto was an Italian economist who resolved that a majority of the wealth resides in just a few elite or upper class. In relation to a process, this means a few causes account for most of the cost (or variation). This prioritizes the "vital few" from the "trivial many" in order to more effectively solve problems.

POISSON DISTRIBUTION: Another discrete probability distribution for attributes data used as an approximation to the binomial. It can be used when $P < 0.1$ and $NP \leq 5$. It is the basis for C charts using attributes data.

PROCESS CONTROL: Defined as having a process behave under an expected frequency of occurrence or within the limits which have been statistically derived. It is a state in which all the points fall in and around the average in a random manner and very few of these approach the limits of the distribution.

RANDOMNESS: The state of collecting individual data values without any expected frequency or basis, yet they may become defined once a distribution is perceived.

RANGE: The difference between the minimum and maximum score.

SAMPLE: A known quantity designated by (n) or the size of the sample. It is randomly pulled from a population parameter in order to provide statistical data.

SPECIAL CAUSE: A cause which is attributable to some assignable item off the x axis of a control chart. Special causes are assignable causes such as people, machine, materials, etc.

SPECIFICATION: Quality specs or product specs; set by engineering or determined by the demands of the customer, keeping in mind Deming's philosophy—"The customer is King."

SPREAD: The variability existing in a distribution of data; can also be thought of as the dispersion of data around the measures of central tendency such as the mean.

STABLE PROCESS: A process that is under statistical control as well as lacking in assignable or special causes of variation.

STANDARD DEVIATION: The main statistic to measure the spread or dispersion of a distribution or of a process when applied with the use of control charts.

STATISTICS: Information derived from a sampled population. The information is arranged in such a manner as to make interpretation of the data easy and to infer something about the population from the sample which has been randomly drawn.

STUDENT'S t DISTRIBUTION: Used when the sample size is less than 50 and required wehn n < 30 or the variance of the distribution is unknown; compensates for smaller sample sizes and is used primarily for mean comparisons or process capability studies.

VARIABLE DATA: Continuous data obtainable via measurable results such as dimensional data (heights, widths) or electrical data (resistance, current).

VARIATION: The degree of change in the spread of a distribution of scores. Many things built by man or by nature have some inherent natural variability. This variation shows up graphically in a distribution of scores.

Acknowledgments

The author gives special thanks to Jean LaDouceur for her contribution to the validation section of this chapter and her biotechnical expertise and assistance, and owes acknowledgment to my immediate circle of friends, colleagues, and family for providing support and encouragement during the development of this chapter.

References

[1]   Ishikawa, K. *Guide to Quality Control.* Nordica International Limited, 1976.

[2]   Taylor, J.K. *Quality Assurance of Chemical Measurements.* Lewis, 1982.

[3]   Young, H.D. *Statistical Treatment of Experimental Data.* McGraw-Hill, 1962.

[4]   Tanis, E.A.*Statistics II: Estimation and TEsts of Hypotheses.* Harcourt Brace Jovanovich, 1987.

[5]   Grant, E.L. and Leavenworth, R.S. *Statistical Quality Control.* McGraw-Hill, 1980.

[6]   Title 21, Code of Federal Regulations.Washington, DC: Office of the Federal Register, National Archives and Records Administration, 1989.

[7]   *Statistics for Experimenters.* Box, Hunter and Hunter.

[8]   Swartz, G. "Analysis of Variance Factorial Design." *Applied Data Analysis, Module III.* Swartz and Associates, 1988.

[9]   Jung, C.G. *The Undiscovered Self.* The New American Library, 1958.

[10]   "Biological Tests/Design and Analysis of Biological Assays <III>." *USP XXI.*

[11]   Levin, R.I. *Statistics for Management.* Prentice-Hall, 1984.

8 Environmental and safety programs for biotechnology

M. Sigourney

Contents

8.1 Safety and waste management

Environmental, health, and safety (EHS) concerns should be an important aspect of any quality assurance (QA) program. In some biotechnology companies, "Environment, Health, and Safety" is a separate department, reporting directly to the president or CEO. In many smaller companies, however, EHS is housed under facilities, human resources, or QA departments. Regardless of the administrative system employed, the basic purpose and functions of an EHS program are fairly universal throughout the biotechnology industry.

The assurance of safe working conditions for the employee and protection of the facility and community environments are integral components of responsible facility operation. Providing a safe and healthy work environment not only helps assure high worker morale but also promotes efficient facility operation. Good quality control (QC) and a high level of product uniformity are more easily attained when safe working conditions are maintained. An active EHS program also helps assist a company in meeting regulatory requirements imposed by local, state, or federal agencies. Most regulatory agencies are very willing to assist a company in meeting regulatory requirements if the company has illustrated "good intent" by establishing and supporting an EHS program. Companies which have made no attempt to develop such policies or programs usually find the cost of regulatory noncompliance financially devastating.

An effective EHS program requires solid corporate commitment to succeed. Financial resources and sufficient manpower must be dedicated to developing and maintaining a program. Personnel must be trained initially and provided with opportunities to update their training annually. Basic equipment such as first aid kits, eyewash and safety shower stations, alarm systems, and spill response supplies must be purchased and maintained.

The total cost in supplies and manpower is a very small component of an annual corporate operating budget, but without these designated commitments, an effective EHS program is impossible. The costs involved in setting up a safety program are more than compensated for in terms of improved employee morale, lower accident and absenteeism rates, and, in many cases, reduced insurance costs. Beyond these financial benefits are the regulatory "hammers" wielded by federal, state and local authorities. Failure to provide adequate employee training, to obtain appropriate facility permits and licensing, and to properly dispose of hazardous wastes all carry fines and penalties which can effectively bankrupt a facility. Even the suggestion of unsafe working conditions or lack of corporate concern for the environment can devastate sales of a company trying to compete in the public marketplace.

8.2 Setting up the program

8.2.1 The "corporate blessing"

An effective EHS program must have official recognition and the corporate blessing if it is to survive. A policy statement from the president or CEO should be included in the employee handbook, safety manual, or other official company document. The program must be publicly sanctioned by management, and EHS concerns should be considered in any corporate decision making, whether in regard to a new product, a facility expansion, or a change in in-house procedures.

8.2.2 Program Administrator

The EHS program needs a focal figure for effective administration. This individual may be the facility manager, quality director, safety coordinator, EHS committee chair or any other designated employee. Regardless of title, this individual should be clearly identified to both management and the employees. This focal figure is usually responsible for handling/coordinating the routine elements of the safety program: training, documentation, and interaction with regulatory agencies.

Most biotechnology companies have developed some type of on-site safety committee which usually oversees the EHS program and functions as a critical communication link between management and employees. Facilities handling radioactivity are required to have a radiation safety committee, and often this committee is expanded to address other safety and health concerns as well.

8.2.3 The Committee

The committee is usually composed of representatives from management and all departments in the facility. Most members should be management-level employees; this emphasizes the commitment of management to safety and ensures that recommended actions will have the financial and signatory authority to be implemented. It is also crucial to have nonmanagement representation on the committee. Technical-level employees are very involved with day-to-day operations and can provide valuable input about the needs and concerns of employees, as well as technical expertise. Often, technical-level committee memberships are rotating positions with one- or two-year terms. Companies with an active safety program have found that positions on the safety committee are coveted and competition for membership is keen.

In very large companies, it may be necessary to have several EHS committees, each representing a specific department or location within the company. Regardless of size, it is crucial that effective two-way communication be maintained between management and employees.

8.2.4 The Committee Role

The responsibilities of the safety committee cross all departmental boundaries. The safety committee:

1. Develops environmental health and safety policies;
2. Monitors compliance with these policies, usually through facility audits;
3. Develops and monitors employee training (may be delegated to an in-house trainer, area managers, or an outside consultant);
4. Monitors compliance with federal, state and local regulations (possibly in conjunction with the facility's regulatory affairs office);
5. Reviews and investigates accident reports; and
6. Advises management on the EHS status of the facility and upcoming changes which may impact the company.

In many companies, the focal figure for the program or another member of the safety committee may be designated to handle specific tasks, including the preparation of regulatory submissions and interfacing with regulatory agencies. In other companies, this may be handled directly by regulatory affairs.

In most situations, the safety manager and safety committee serve as advisory personnel in the facility. They should review procedures and operations in the laboratories and other parts of the facility and advise area managers of specific problems or suggested changes. The safety committee should be viewed not as corporate police, but as safety counselors. Of course, if a situation arises where immediate action is necessary, the committee or safety manager should have the authority to take action at once. It is advisable in the majority of situations, however, to work with an area manager or supervisor to correct a problem. This provides for a consistent chain of command for employees and assures much better cooperation between managers and the safety committee.

8.2.5 Documentation

A set of written procedures and guidelines is very important for an effective program. Most companies develop a safety manual or directory, while others may include safety precautions or procedures as part of their standard operating procedures (SOPs). Regardless of how the information is distributed, it is vital that all employees know and understand the proper safety procedures to follow in any job situation.

Reports from the safety committee, meeting minutes, and audit/inspection summaries are vital communications. Management and employees need to keep informed about the status of their company. The State of California has recently enacted legislation (SB 198) requiring the development of a written Injury Prevention Plan (IPP), which consists of a written safety program and consistent, effective communication concerning safety and health issues.

Some facilities have found that a monthly safety newsletter can be both informative and entertaining. Health and safety news is often eagerly received if presented with a light (or humorous) touch. Tongue-in-cheek quizzes, crossword puzzles, and riddles covering topics as dry as regulatory agencies, toxicology, and radiation inspections can keep employees informed and enthusiastic about safety.

8.3 The paper trail

Documentation is an essential part of every EHS program. Written reports are required by regulatory agencies at all levels. Smaller companies may have to report only on hazardous waste disposal, chemical inventories, and emergency response procedures. Companies which have air emissions, discharges to sewers or holding tanks, threshold quantities of hazardous materials, or other regulated activities may find that monthly or quarterly report filings require hundreds of man-hours. This text will highlight some of the regulatory agencies and waste handling requirements.

State and local agencies may have extensive reporting requirements that cannot be addressed here. Every facility must determine under which agencies and regulations it is administered and comply with those specific requirements. It is very important to bear in mind that regulations tend to change very rapidly. A corollary to Murphy's Law should be: No law changes faster than the one you aren't watching!

With all of the different agencies and levels of government involved in regulating biotechnology facilities, it is vital to keep in touch with several reliable resources: newsletters, the Federal Register, industrial trade journals, and legislative consultants. Ignorance of the law is not only dangerous—it can be financially devastating.

8.4   The Regulatory Jungle

EHS areas are regulated by agencies at all governmental levels. Federal regulations pre-empt any state or local statutes, unless the state or local statutes are more restrictive.

8.4.1   The federal agencies

The primary federal regulatory agency involved with employee health and safety is the Occupational Safety and Health Administration (OSHA). Other federal agencies that impact safety and the environment include the Environmental Protection Agency (EPA), Department of Transportation (DOT), the Food and Drug Administration (FDA), and the Nuclear Regulatory Commission (NRC). These five federal agencies—and their state/local counterparts—impact the majority of business and operational functions in the biotechnology industry.

8.4.1.1   OSHA

OSHA was formed in 1970 to "assure safe and healthful working conditions for every man and woman in the nation." Safety regulations developed and enforced under OSHA include stipulations for the handling and labeling of hazardous materials used in the workplace and specific requirements for equipment/machinery guarding. Health regulations are exemplified by employee health monitoring requirements and the establishment of exposure limits for hazardous materials and maximum contaminant levels for workplace air. Specific guidelines and requirements under OSHA will be discussed in detail in the sections dealing with biohazardous materials and chemical safety.

8.4.1.2   EPA

The EPA is charged with setting federal air and water standards that are enforced by state and local agencies. In addition, the EPA regulates the handling and disposal of chemical and other hazardous wastes. This function of the EPA is carried out primarily through the Resource Conservation and Recovery Act (RCRA) and the Superfund Amendments and Reauthorization Act of 1986 (SARA).

The RCRA was passed in 1976 to deal with municipal and hazardous waste problems and to encourage conservation and recycling of natural resources. RCRA has established a "cradle-to-grave" management system for hazardous wastes, promoting recycling where possible and assuring proper disposal of nonrecyclable wastes. A nationwide system of chemical waste manifesting, in conjunction with a permit system for waste generators and treatment, storage, and disposal facilities (TSDFs), has been established to track chemical wastes.

SARA is an extension of earlier legislation (CERCLA, the Comprehensive Environmental Response, Compensation and Liability Act) designed to identify and clean up chemical and hazardous substance releases into any part of the environment.

Title III, a stand-alone section of SARA, has particular significance for the biotechnology industry. Contained within Title III are requirements for emergency/contingency planning in the event of hazardous materials releases. The community right-to-know sections of SARA III require that owners or operators of facilities provide information on the storage, handling, and use of hazardous materials within their facilities. This information must be provided to state agencies, local emergency responders, and, with the exception of trade secrets, to the general public. Planned or accidental releases of restricted materials into the environment must be reported to specified agencies within a designated time frame.

8.4.1.3 DOT

The DOT oversees the movement of hazardous materials and hazardous wastes over any public road. All hazardous material or waste must be shipped in DOT-approved containers in properly placarded vehicles. Hazardous wastes may be transported only by licensed hazardous waste haulers. All shipments must be properly labeled and manifested from the site of origin to the final destination.

8.4.1.4 FDA

The role of the FDA is perhaps most well-known to regulatory affairs and quality control managers. This federal agency and its impact on biotechnology is addressed in other sections of this book.

8.4.1.5 NRC

The NRC sets federal standards for the handling of radioactive materials and wastes. Over half of the fifty states have entered into agreements with the NRC to accept authority for by-products, sources, and small amounts of specific low-level radioactive materials produced or used in that state. Those states having agreements with the NRC have developed state requirements with regard to handling and disposal of radioactivity. Each "agreement state" sets its own require-ments regarding the licensing of facilities to possess radioactive materials, as well as specific handling and disposal procedures. Nonagreement states rely on the NRC to license and inspect all facilities handling radioactive materials or wastes in those states.

8.4.2 State agencies

Many states have developed a regulatory framework parallel to that in place at the federal level. Employee safety and health programs are administered through state labor and industrial relations departments, OSHAs, or human resource boards. State health services and toxics departments develop and administer programs specific to health, hazardous materials handling/ disposal, and emergency response programs. Usually the development and enforcement of air and water standards is done at the county or regional board level.

8.4.3 Local agencies

Cities have also developed specific policies with regard to EHS. City or county planning commissions regulate facility siting and develop specific zoning restrictions. Business licenses and permits for hazardous materials handling and storage are also issued at the local level.

In recent years, many cities and local planning regions have become very restrictive with regard to the types of hazardous materials they will permit within their jurisdictional boundaries. Those areas which do permit the handling of hazardous materials are requiring facilities using these materials to utilize the best available technology to minimize the potential for community exposure.

Daily monitoring of air emissions and waste water discharges is required in many areas. Quarterly or annual reports are frequently required by local air and water boards to ascertain the quantity of materials being released into the environment. In addition, businesses in many areas are required to report any release or threatened release of a hazardous material to the environment. Not only must emergency responders—fire, police, and medical personnel—be notified, but local and state environmental agencies as well.

Local fire districts have always been responsible for facility inspections to determine compliance with fire codes. In recent years, however, local fire marshals and inspectors have become more closely involved with hazardous materials handling and storage as well. The *Uniform Fire Code* and the *Uniform Building Code* were revised in 1988 to reflect the concerns of fire and building inspectors with regard to hazardous materials. The *Uniform Fire Code* section on hazardous materials (Article 80) was expanded from six pages to fifty. Specific requirements for container construction, sprinkler types and number, wall construction, secondary containment, and maximum storage quantities of "haz mats" are identified. These codes are industry standards and will be adopted in whole or in part by most fire protection districts in the United States. Compliance with these code requirements will be mandatory for any business handling hazardous materials.

Local fire inspectors may make additional requests for safety equipment specific to a given industry. For example, biotechnology facilities in the San Francisco Bay Area have been requested to use metal containers with close-fitting lids as secondary containment vessels for the collection of biohazardous/infectious wastes rather than using plastic containers; metal signs, rather than plastic, are required for posting radiation and biological hazards.

Special hazardous materials permits are also required by local fire marshals. These permits are often specific for the materials used, and fees may be pro-rated based on the quantity and classification of hazardous materials handled. Such permitting is required in addition to any state or federal permits for hazardous materials handling and hazardous waste generation.

Table 8.1 "Who's Who" of Regulatory Agencies

ACTIVITY	FEDERAL	STATE	LOCAL
Product Purity/Licensing	FDA	Health	—
Worker Health/Safety	OSHA	"OSHA"/Labor	Fire/Health
Haz Mat Handling	EPA/OSHA	Health	Fire/Health
Haz Mat Storage	EPA	Health/Toxics	Fire
Waste Transport	DOT	Highway Patrol	Fire/Public Works
Waste Disposal	EPA (RCRA)	Health/Toxics	Health
Emergency Planning	EPA (SARA)	Health	Health
Biologicals	OSHA/EPA CDC	Health	Health
Air Standards	EPA	Regional Air Bd	Local Air Bd
Water Standards	EPA	Regional Water Bd	Local Water Bd

8.5 Emergency response/evacuation planning

Federal legislation has mandated a program for emergency planning and response to hazardous materials spills/releases under SARA Title III (40 CFR 300-313). This legislation is also known as the Emergency Planning and Community Right to Know Amendment (EPCRA). Title III is divided into several sections; sections 301–303 require that every state develop a network of local and regional planning groups which can mobilize an emergency response to natural disasters and hazardous materials incidents. This network expands further, and in most states local planning areas require private industry to develop emergency response programs for their own facilities. The format for these emergency or "business" plans is specified by the local administering agency, which may be the county, city, or other "special district."

8.6 Other required reports

Other sections of SARA III (311–312) require that businesses handling listed chemicals above specified "threshold quantities" must report these chemicals, their hazard classifications, and the actual quantities handled on site.

State and local agencies may also require facilities to report the hazardous materials they handle. In many situations, the chemicals specified by federal requirements are not the same as those specified by state or local authorities. This dichotomy often requires the facilities to file separate reports for federal, state, and local agencies.

There have been attempts to reduce and simplify some of the required reporting. For example, California has made agreements with the federal government to incorporate some of the SARA-required information into its state-mandated business plans. (These plans address emergency response procedures to be taken by a facility in the event of spills, unplanned chemical releases, or other disasters.) Even with this simplification, there is still a great deal of paperwork involved for these required reports.

8.7 Key elements

Several key administrative elements must be addressed by every biotechnology facility to comply with required regulatory reporting. If these elements are carefully prepared and updated on a regular basis, the data required by most regulatory agencies can be accessed with a minimum of difficulty.

8.7.1 Chemical inventory

A chemical inventory is required by almost every regulatory agency. If records have not been adequately maintained to date, a complete facility inventory will probably be necessary. The most efficient, although time-consuming, procedure for doing this is usually a physical room-by-room inventory. When the physical inventory is completed, the data must be sorted and compiled. This is most easily done using a computer spreadsheet. If the facility has a computer network, this system may be input to a network-wide data base.

All computer systems have some type of spreadsheet format, and most can be adapted easily for inventory control data. Before beginning any inventory procedures, it is advisable to determine what types of information may need to be retrieved from the system. This should help assure that the information will be properly collected and sorted, initially, and help prevent the need to reinventory or reformat later.

SARA requires chemical name, hazard classification, storage (container) type, CAS (chemical abstract service) number, DOT number, and location within the facility of each listed chemical. This information can be retrieved from most spreadsheets if the data is entered in a row/column configuration such as that below.

CHEMICAL	HAZARD CLASS	LOCATIONS		CAS NO.	DOT NO.
		Lab 2	Room 3		
Acetonitrile	FL, Toxic	2 x 4 Lit.	1 Lit.	75-05-8	NA 1648

This system easily accommodates changes in the data base and may be sorted by location, hazard class, chemical, etc. The inventory can be updated by monitoring incoming materials through the shipping/receiving department and spent materials through the user departments.

8.7.2 Maps

Maps and diagrams of the physical plant are essential, both for daily operations within the facility and for reporting compliance. Site maps with roads, hydrants, and emergency equipment are usually requested by every fire protection district. In addition, the location of chemical handling and storage areas should be indicated on a second map. Floor drains, sewer lines, and gas mains should be indicated on a third set of maps.

8.7.3 Communications

All emergency response plans and business plans must indicate how employees and emergency responders will be alerted to an emergency or hazardous material release. These procedures should be clearly posted within the facility and made part of standard employee training. Companies are also required to have a means of notifying the surrounding community in the event of a hazardous material release that could impact the community in any way. (Among the "haz mat" incidents that could impact a community are: chemical runoff to a storm sewer, a spill in the company parking lot that could spread outside the facility, or a fume or "toxic cloud" release.)

8.7.4 Contingency plans

Every facility must have a procedure in place for response to a spill of any material handled by that facility. If the facility does not have personnel properly trained and equipped to contain and clean up the spill, arrangements should be made with a private contractor to handle any spill which may occur. These arrangements should be made before an emergency situation arises. If community emergency responders—police, highway patrol, or fire department—are required to clean up a spill, the facility responsible for the incident will be billed for the cleanup, in addition to any fines which may be imposed.

8.8   Emergency response teams/programs

Many facilities have developed emergency response teams (ERTs) to deal with medical, spill, and other emergencies. Having an ERT helps assure rapid response to most emergency situations and illustrates the commitment of management to the health and safety of its employees. The development of an ERT requires a long-term commitment by management, and requires planning and assured financial resources for the program.

An ERT is usually composed of spill responders and medical responders; in many situations, the same personnel handle both responsibilities. The ERT must have professional training and the proper equipment for dealing with the emergencies to which it may respond. The responders and other employees must know the limits of the team and never attempt to address an emergency beyond their capabilities.

Federal OSHA has issued specific regulations for the training and management of emergency response teams (29 CFR 1910.120). If team members are required to use respirators during a spill cleanup, additional requirements for respirator users must be met (29 CFR 1910.134). A written respirator program is required for any facility where respirators are in use either on a regular basis or for emergency response only. Respirator users must be properly trained and medically certified to use a respirator. The respirator user's medical status should be reviewed periodically (for instance, annually). Federal regulations and the *NIOSH Guide to Industrial Respiratory Protection* should be consulted before initiating an ERT program.

Emergency medical responders must be trained to handle standard medical emergencies. At a minimum, the medical responder should be CPR-certified and trained in basic first aid. Advanced courses in hazardous materials medical response may be available within the community or through state or local colleges and are recommended if the facility handles hazardous materials. (The University of California, Davis, Hazardous Materials Management Program offers courses in Medical Management of Hazardous Materials Incidents.) Drills and regular training sessions are essential to assure that team members are able to function quickly and efficiently in the event of an emergency.

8.9   Chemical handling and disposal

When developing a program for handling and disposal of chemicals, it is important to be familiar with all of the regulatory agencies that oversee chemical handling. The two lead agencies in this area are OSHA and the Environmental Protection Agency.

8.9.1   The Hazard Communication Standard

OSHA has set federal standards for worker protection with regard to workplace hazards. The Hazard Communication Standard (29 CFR 1910.1200) specifies how employers must alert employees to chemical hazards in the workplace.

1. Employers must establish a written comprehensive Hazard Communication Program, which includes provisions for container labeling, Material Safety Data Sheets (MSDS), and employee training. The written program must be available to all employees and must specify individuals who have responsibility for maintaining MSDS and carrying out training programs.

2. An inventory of hazardous materials in the workplace must be maintained and made available to employees. MSDS for each hazardous material must be available and easily accessible to all employees.

3. All containers of hazardous material must be properly labelled with the name, hazard classification of the material, and specific handling precautions, if applicable.

4. The employer must establish and maintain a training program for all employees who handle or may be exposed to hazardous materials in the workplace. This training may include clerical and business personnel, in addition to laboratory and warehouse employees.

The Federal Hazard Communication Standard has very specific requirements for each of these areas; written documentation of the program is required.

8.9.2   Hazardous waste

Chemicals that are no longer usable by the facility and have certain characteristics such as flammability, toxicity, corrosivity, or reactivity may be defined as "hazardous wastes." Federal and state definitions of hazardous waste may differ, depending on the chemical.

Facilities that generate hazardous wastes must register with the EPA and obtain an identification number. Annual reports must be filed with the EPA and state agencies, as required. In some states, such as California, a state agency may administer some or all of the EPA permits and reporting.

Hazardous wastes must be handled in accordance with both federal and state requirements. These wastes must be accumulated in specified containers in secure areas and may not be held on-site longer than a specified number of days. Accumulation times set by the EPA (federal limits) are listed under 40 CFR 262.34. State agencies may be more restrictive in accumulation times.

Employees who handle any hazardous wastes must be properly trained in appropriate handling techniques, emergency response procedures, and spill remediation, in addition to chemical safety training required under the Hazard Communication Standard.

In many areas, state and local permits and licenses are required to handle and store hazardous materials and to generate hazardous wastes.

8.9.3   Hazardous waste disposal

Until the early 1980s, hazardous chemical wastes were routinely buried at Class I landfills, injected into deep wells, or (illegally) included in municipal landfills. Disposal of hazardous wastes has become much more controlled with the implementation of the so-called "land ban restrictions" included in the RCRA (40 CFR 268.10-268.31).

The "land ban" prohibits the disposal of solvents and certain other specified wastes to any landfill. This prohibition essentially requires that solvent wastes are either recycled or incinerated. The costs of incineration have risen astronomically in recent years and will continue to rise. There are only a handful of hazardous waste incinerators in the United States, and there is little likelihood that many additional sites will be permitted by the EPA, due to environmental concerns over air quality and disposal of incinerator ash, and the unwillingness of most communities to allow these incinerators to be sited nearby.

Solvent recycling is gaining popularity, but most recyclers require a guaranteed volume of a uniform wastestream before they will contract to handle a facility's waste solvents. Most biotechnology facilities do not have large uniform quantities of solvent waste, which makes recycling somewhat difficult. A number of states have developed directories of recyclers and processors to assist companies in recycling their wastes. Additionally, there are often tax incentives for companies which recycle their wastes rather than incinerate them.

The most desirable way to reduce hazardous waste costs is to reduce the amount of hazardous waste generated. Any procedure which generates a wastestream (i.e., HPLC purifications, DNA synthesis, or organic solvent distillation) should be reviewed to determine if the amount of waste solvent can be reduced. If techniques can be altered, materials substituted, or byproduct wastes reused in the process, the amount of hazardous waste and subsequent cost of waste disposal can be reduced. This type of waste minimization is required under RCRA; every generator must indicate on its hazardous waste manifest that a waste minimization program is in effect in its facility.

In California, the Department of Health Services' Alternative Technologies Division has established a grant program available to companies wishing to implement pilot programs for hazardous waste reduction. Other states may have similar programs available.

8.9.4 Hazardous waste transport

Hazardous wastes may only be transported on public roads by licensed hazardous waste haulers. The shipment of any hazardous waste requires proper documentation prior to shipping. A completed "Uniform Waste Manifest" for hazardous waste must be completed and signed by the generator. In some situations, a transporter or waste hauler may include the preparation of shipping papers as part of a packaged service to its customers. Regardless of who completes the forms, the responsibility (and liability) for the shipment of the hazardous waste rests with the generator. The generators must be sure that the manifest properly lists the contents, hazard classifications, and emergency information required for their shipment.

Disposal of hazardous wastes may be done only by licensed TSDFs. Waste generators must be certain that their hazardous wastes arrive at their intended destination. The manifest tracking system requires that shipping papers be returned to the generator from the final TSDF. If paperwork is delayed or incomplete, the generator must follow-up with the transporter or TSDF to ensure that its wastes were properly transported and received. In recent years, barrels (and truckloads) of hazardous wastes have been abandoned by "midnight dumpers" posing as certified haulers. If a hauler offers shipping or disposal rates that seem too good to be true, they usually are.

8.10 Biological materials

The 1980s ushered in a new industry: biotechnology. Prior to the '80s, the environmental health and safety concerns of industry dealt primarily with chemical and radioisotope handling and disposal. Clinical labs and hospitals had always dealt with blood and "human source material," but the introduction of recombinant DNA, coupled with identification of the human immunodeficiency virus (HIV), has made "biologicals" the safety concern of the 1990s.

8.10.1 Recombinant DNA

Recombinant DNA has been strictly regulated by the federal government from the beginning of the biotechnology era. The National Institutes of Health (NIH) in 1983 issued "Guidelines for Research Involving Recombinant DNA Molecules" (*Federal Register*, 48, No. 106, pp. 24556–24581). These guidelines identified specific microorganisms and their hazard classifications and outlined the containment and handling procedures required for each. The guidelines are still considered the definitive regulatory document for recombinant DNA research.

Appendix K of the NIH guidelines addresses large-scale uses of organisms containing recombinant DNA molecules. Any cultures involving greater than ten liters of media must follow the containment and operating procedures set forth in Appendix K. Inactivation of the culture, filtration of exhaust gases, emergency procedures, and other safety specifications are clearly designated for each of three containment levels.

8.10.2 Human source material

Of more widespread concern to the biotechnology industry has been the handling and disposal of human source materials. Blood and other body fluids are processed daily by thousands of clinicians, researchers, and technicians. The prevalence of hepatitis B and HIV in many of these samples has caused universal concern and resulted in legislation at both the state and federal levels.

Until the late 1980s, human source material and medical or infectious waste was controlled primarily by local health departments. Some states, such as California, had legislation addressing "infectious waste," but clear definitions and specific guidelines were needed. Federal OSHA drafted a document in 1989 entitled "Bloodborne Pathogens," which was aimed at protecting individuals who could be potentially exposed to human source materials in the workplace. In 1991, this draft document was adopted and became law (29 CRF 1910.1030). The Bloodborne Pathogens regulations are now enforceable under OSHA. The EPA has drafted "Standards for Tracking and Management of Medical Waste", an interim final rule (*Federal Register*, Vol. 54, No. 56, pp. 12326–12395). These two federal documents and legislation developing in states throughout the nation have dramatically changed the handling of human source material for many companies and institutions.

8.10.3 Disposal

Documentation procedures for the disposal of biohazardous waste may vary with state and local agencies, but some form of in-house recordkeeping for these wastes is required.
Validation records and temperature control charts for steam sterilizers are required for manufacturers under Good Manufacturing Practices (GMP); autoclaves used for deactivating wastes also must have temperature records for each run. Every bag of waste processed in-house must be traceable as well. Many companies number each bag with a date and location code, then attach an indicator strip to each bag for temperature verification. Monthly autoclave challenges using a biological indicator or other approved test are also required.

Materials transported off-site for disposal must be tracked. Transporters of biohazardous/infectious waste must be selected with the same criteria used for chemical waste transporters. The ultimate disposal of each shipment must be documented in some verifiable manner. Medical waste generators are being held legally responsible for their wastes in the same manner that chemical waste generators have been.

Just as with chemical hazardous wastes, a manifest tracking system may be the most efficient means of tracking biological/infectious wastes. This system has been instituted in three eastern states under the interim rule set by the EPA in 1989. This system may be adopted by the EPA for implementation across the United States, or individual states may choose to develop their own medical waste tracking systems. In either situation, biotechnology facilities must plan to implement a thorough tracking system for their biological/infectious wastes in the immediate future if they do not already have effective tracking systems in place. The system must be able to identify the source of the wastes, the inactivation procedures used, if any, and the final disposal site of the materials. Any inactivation procedures used must be validated for effectiveness and records of equipment maintenance and validation records retained for at least three years.

8.10.4 Employee protection

Federal OSHA has adopted the bulk of the Centers for Disease Control Guidelines for handling infectious/biological materials. Any employee who handles or may handle human source material, or who may be exposed to human source materials as a part of his required work duties, must be properly trained. Under the Bloodborne Pathogens rule, every employment position must be evaluated in terms of the possibility for exposure to potentially infectious materials. Any individual working in a position where exposure may occur, even if it is only once per month, must be properly trained in the appropriate techniques for handling, infection control, and proper disposal of infectious materials.

Employees must be provided with the appropriate personal protective equipment needed for their work environment. Gloves, safety glasses or full face shields, face masks, or respirators, gowns, lab aprons, or other necessary equipment must be provided by the employer. Each individual also must participate in documented training in the use of this protective equipment. Such training and documentation is comparable to other "right-to-know" requirements covered under the Hazard Communication Standard of Federal OSHA.

8.10.5 Medical tracking/prophylaxis

If individuals may be exposed to human source materials or other pathogenic materials, appropriate training must be provided regarding the potential for exposure to these infectious pathogens. Medical tracking may be required for these employees, as well as specific vaccination programs. Hepatitis B vaccinations must be made available at no cost to employees who may be exposed to human patient samples, bulk human serum, infectious wastes, or other areas where human source material may be encountered. When vaccines for hepatitis C and HIV are available, employers no doubt will be required to provide these vaccinations for employees as well.

Some companies require vaccinations prior to employee placement in some high-risk assignments such as cell culture labs. If vaccinations are not required but a position may involve exposure to human source materials, the employee may refuse to participate in a vaccination program. The employer is cautioned, however, to document the fact that the individual was informed of the company's infection control policies and the company's offer to provide the vaccination(s) to the employee. Records of participation in the vaccination program or refusal to participate must be documented. Employees who initially decline to participate in the vaccination program may opt to participate later at no cost to the employee.

8.10.6 Written infection control program

Every company handling human source materials should have written procedures for handling biological materials. At a minimum, the procedures should outline specific handling procedures, personal protective equipment, and spill control procedures. Emergency response procedures must also be clearly defined, including procedures to be taken in the event of overt employee exposure to potentially infectious materials. Needlesticks, splashes, inhalation of potentially infectious aerosols, or other possible exposures must be identified as incidents requiring medical attention. Company procedures must identify steps that will be taken to medically assist the employee, identify the source and exposure potential of the contaminating material, and procedures necessary to protect others from further exposures.

8.11 Where to find regulatory information

As mentioned previously, every state and community has its own set of regulations controlling worker health and community safety. An abbreviated summary of the key federal regulations discussed in this chapter is provided as a brief overview of where to begin in the regulatory jungle. This list is by no means exhaustive, but the major areas of concern to biotechnology companies are identified. Each state has its own set of regulations, as well, which may be more restrictive than federal requirements. Be certain to check with state and local codes and regulations before implementing programs or procedures concerning employee training, waste disposal, materials handling, or record keeping.

CODE OF FEDERAL REGISTER CITATIONS

"Employee Right-to-Know"	29 CFR 1910.1200
Hazardous Waste Handling	40 CFR 264.16
Bloodborne Pathogens	29 CFR 1910.1030
Emergency Response Teams	29 CFR 1910.120
Respirator Usage	29 CFR 1910.134
Hazardous Waste Accumulation	40 CFR 262.34
Hazardous Waste Transport	
(shipping and packaging)	49 CFR 173
Hazardous Waste Manifesting	49 CFR 172.205
	40 CFR 262.20
Chemical (DOT) Classifications	49 CFR 172.101–2
"Land Bans"	40 CFR 268.10–31
Chemical Inventories (CERCLA/SARA)	40 CFR 306
Emergency Planning and Notification	40 CFR 355

References

[1] EPA Title III Fact Sheet. Washington, DC: United States Environmental Protection Agency, August 1988.

[2] *EPA Guide for Infectious Waste Management.* (EPA/530-SW-86-014) Washington, DC: United States Environmental Protection Agency, Office of Solid Waste and Emergency Response. (Available through National Technical Information Service, Springfield, VA 22161 (PB86-199130)).

[3] Bollinger, N.J. and Schutz, R.H. *NIOSH Guide to Industrial Respiratory Protection.* 1987. U.S. Department of Health and Human Services, Public Health Service, NIOSH, 4676 Columbia Parkway, Cincinnati, OH 45226.

[4] Miller, Brinton M. et al. *Laboratory Safety: Principles and Practices.* Washington, DC: American Society for Microbiology, 1986.,

[5] *Biosafety in Microbiological and Biomedical Laboratories.* HHS Publication No. (CDC) 88-8395. U.S. Department of Health and Human Services, Public Health Service, National Institutes of Health, Bethesda, MD 20892.

[6] *Protection of Laboratory Workers from Infectious Disease Transmitted by Blood and Tissue.* NCCLS Document M29-P (Vol. 7, No. 9). National Committee for Clinical Laboratory Standards, 771 East Lancaster Avenue, Villanova, PA 19085.

[7] *California Waste Exchange: A Newsletter/Catalog.* State Department of Health Services, Alternative Technology Division, 744 P Street, P.O. Box 942732, Sacramento, CA 94234-7320.

[8] Hazardous Chemical "List of Lists." Office of Hazardous Materials Data Management, Environmental Affairs Agency, P.O. Box 2815, Sacramento, CA 95812.

[9] "California's Biotechnology Permits and Regulations—A Description." Interagency Task Force on Biotechnology, State of California, 1986.

[10] Title 29, Code of Federal Regulations, Sections 1900–1910. Washington, DC: Office of the Federal Register, National Archives and Records Administration.

[11] Title 40, Code of Federal Regulations, Sections 190–399. Washington, DC: Office of the Federal Register, National Archives and Records Administration.

[12] Title 49, Code of Federal Regulations, Sections 100–177. Washington, DC: Office of the Federal Register, National Archives and Records Administration.

[13] Title 22.1, California Regulatory Code.

9 Regulatory issues—United States

C. L. Spencer

Contents

9.1 Introduction

The procedural aspects of regulatory affairs can be quite technical. However, to deal effectively with the details, there needs first to be an understanding of regulatory affairs in the broader perspective. The goal of this chapter is to provide a more conceptual approach to product development and regulatory affairs rather than reciting regulations or offering a "how-to" manual. Its scope is limited to functions of the United States Food and Drug Administration (FDA) and their application of the Food Drug & Cosmetic Act (FD&CA) [1] and the Public Health Service (PHS) Act [2]. These are two of the primary laws FDA uses to regulate drugs and devices, including products derived from biotechnology. Although biotechnology has its nuances, it basically is just a variation of manufacturing technology. Thus, the same rules that apply to other drug and device products also apply to products derived from biotechnology.

There are other laws and agencies applicable to the development and marketing of biotechnology derived products. Some of these may be discussed in other chapters of this text.

9.2 Regulatory affairs

When development of a product is undertaken, usually some form of a project team is assembled. The team should consist of various disciplines to include research, product development, manufacturing, quality assurance (QA), marketing, finance, and regulatory affairs. Each discipline brings to the forum its own unique skills, experiences, and perspective, which, as part of the team, can be integrated to move a product to market.

The skills and experiences brought to the team by regulatory affairs are varied. The skills should include such things as a working knowledge of administrative law and in particular the laws enforced by FDA, a strong communication and negotiation ability, organization, and an acute attention to detail. The experiences should include familiarity with the division of FDA with jurisdiction over the product and the regulations to be applied during development and marketing.

Equally as important as the skills and experiences, however, is the perspective regulatory affairs must have when working with a product. Regulatory affairs provides the link between science and business—the link which takes the product from the research bench to market. Every member of the project team contributes to this process, but regulatory affairs is in the unique position of compiling all relevant information on the product, presenting it to the FDA, negotiating approval requirements, and assuring legal compliance, all within the guidelines of the business plan. Their responsibility is to make concise, consistent, and persuasive presentations to FDA following the format and procedures required.

FDA generally has one person in each reviewing division who serves as a single point of contact to enable more efficient communications and help avoid misunderstandings. This person is usually referred to as the Consumer Safety Officer (CSO). FDA strongly encourages the designation of one person as a point of contact for the product sponsor. This is the role of regulatory affairs.

9.3 FDA

The FDA is an administrative agency and, like other administrative agencies, was created to deal with problems affecting all citizens (e.g., food and drug supplies in the United States). The powers delegated to FDA by Congress are characteristic of each of the three branches of government: the *legislative* power to issue rules, the *executive* power to investigate, and the *judicial* power to adjudicate.

The FDA is divided into five centers, each of which may have some exposure to the use of biotechnology in the products for which it is responsible:

1. Center for Drug Evaluation and Research,
2. Center for Biologics Evaluation and Research,
3. Center for Devices and Radiological Health,
4. Center for Veterinary Medicine, and
5. Center for Food Safety and Applied Nutrition.

Over the years, these centers have been grouped somewhat differently or referred to by somewhat different titles. Nevertheless, the overall categories for which the FDA is responsible remains consistent.

Since 1938, the FDA has been empowered to evaluate the *safety* of drugs before a product may be marketed. In 1962, the law was amended to require a demonstration of the drug's *effectiveness*, as well. The 1962 amendment further required that such effectiveness be supported by "substantial evidence."

The product sponsor holds the burden of proof of substantial evidence. This means that the party (e.g., product sponsor) carrying the burden will lose if the trier of fact (in this case, the FDA) remains in doubt or is not convinced to the degree required (e.g., by the presentation of substantial evidence).

The concept of substantial evidence is a nebulous one but perhaps can be put into some perspective by comparing it to two other commonly applied burdens of proof. In civil cases, the trier of fact must be convinced by a "preponderance of evidence." In contrast, a trier of fact in a criminal matter must be convinced "beyond a reasonable doubt." Substantial evidence lies somewhere in between these two thresholds, neither of which can be defined with any specificity. It remains the responsibility of the trier of fact (e.g., the FDA) to determine at what point the threshold has been met.

The regulation of drugs and other products by the FDA came about because of problems in the food and drug supplies in the Unites States. It was not possible for the public to adequately protect themselves against products which by their nature carried the possibility of latent defects or dangers—or sometimes, fraud. Therefore, the FDA's focus when applying the substantial evidence test is on protection of the public and not on the product sponsor.

9.4   Rulemaking and adjudication

Rulemaking and adjudication are two important administrative activities of agencies such as the FDA. These and their related terms are defined in the Administrative Procedures Act [3] and can be summarized as follows:

RULEMAKING: The process for formulating, amending, or repealing a rule.

RULE: An agency statement of general or particular applicability and future effect designed to implement, interpret, or prescribe law or policy.

ADJUDICATION: Agency process for the formulation of an order.

ORDER: A final disposition by an agency in a matter other than rulemaking but including licensing.

A useful method of distinguishing between these two activities is by looking to the person(s) affected. Adjudication or orders tend to affect the rights of individuals or classes of individuals. Rulemaking, on the other hand, tends to affect the public and those governed by the rules, such as drug/device manufacturers generally.

Most people are familiar with the process of adjudication as it occurs in response to the submission of information to the FDA for approval to investigate or market a product. The FDA reviews the information submitted and responds to the sponsor with its disposition, or order. The determinations are made on a case-by-case basis.

Rulemaking, by contrast, is characterized generally by a process providing notice and comment by the affected public. When the FDA proposes a new rule, the rule is published in the *Federal Register* to give the public notice of the FDA's intended action. The notice provides for a comment period during which time interested persons may comment to the FDA on the intended action. If the FDA subsequently makes the rule final, either in its original form or modified as a result of comments received, the FDA publishes its response to the comments in what is called the "preamble" to the rule. This process is a lengthy one, which creates a problem for the FDA when it wants to respond quickly to a problem or needs to communicate to others what may be expected of them by the FDA. To resolve this dilemma, the FDA uses two other methods for disseminating information to the regulated public. These are *Guidelines* and *Points to Consider* documents.

9.4.1   *Guidelines* and *Points To Consider*

Guidelines issued by the FDA communicate procedures or standards of general applicability that are acceptable to the FDA. They represent the FDA's formal position on the subject matter upon which a person may rely with assurance that it is acceptable to FDA [4]. They generally cover areas with which the FDA has had significant experience and, thus, sufficient time to develop generally applicable guidance criteria.

Points to Consider are similar to *Guidelines*. However, they are used to communicate information about areas with which the FDA has had little experience (e.g., the development of new technologies such as biotechnology). These generally involve new and rapidly changing areas of information.

In contrast to laws and regulations, *Guidelines* and *Points to Consider* are not legal requirements enforceable, *per se,* by the FDA. Their primary purpose is to provide a mechanism for the FDA to communicate with the regulated public in an informal and expeditious manner. Therefore, they may be challenged where there is a strong scientific basis for so doing.

9.5   United States Pharmacopeia (USP) and National Formulary (NF)

The USP/NF, published on a periodic basis, has as its purpose to provide "authoritative standards and specifications for materials and substances and their preparations that are used in the practice of the healing arts." It "establishes titles, definitions, descriptions, and standards for identity, quality, strength, purity, packaging and labeling, and also, where practicable, bioavailability, stability, procedures for proper handling and storage, and methods for their examination and formulas for their manufacture or preparation" [5].

The USP/NF are recognized as official compendia and are referenced in various statutes as a basis for determining the strength, quality, purity, packaging, and labeling of drugs and related articles. The conformance of an individual product to compendial requirements, however, is a matter of compliance rather than standard setting [6]. Therefore, it is not necessary for a manufacturer to use a USP/NF method to analyze a compendial product. The method used, however, must be of equivalent or higher accuracy, and the product must meet the compendial requirements when tested by the FDA using the USP/NF method. It is recognized that the USP/NF methods were not designed for and are often not the most appropriate methods for use by manufacturers in batch release testing [7].

"Adulterated" and "misbranded" are legal terms of art which encompass a variety of violations possible under the FD&CA. Under certain conditions, a drug or device may be deemed to be adulterated or misbranded if it does not meet the requirements of strength, quality, or purity recognized in an official compendium such as the USP/NF [8].

9.6 Product characterization

As explained previously, the FDA is divided into several centers. Proper characterization of a product is necessary not only to determine the applicable regulations but also the center of the FDA with which one should be working.

As was also mentioned above, the creation of laws and regulations by agencies such as the FDA usually stems from the identification of a specific problem affecting the public on whose behalf the agency is acting to protect. This kind of approach inevitably results in a sort of patchwork quilt effect with laws or regulations that may relate to only one type of product or, in other instances, to many product types.

Similarly, proper characterization of the stage of development or manufacture of a product can have a significant impact on the rigor with which it is regulated. Thus, before one can address the questions of compliance with applicable laws and regulations, the product must be characterized as to its nature (e.g., drug, device, biologic, etc.) and, at the same time, considered as to its stage of development and/or manufacture. "Stage of development" looks at characterization of a product by whether it is pre- or post-approval by the FDA for marketing (e.g., Is it a product in preclinical or clinical testing vs. a product in commercial distribution for sale?). "Stage of manufacture" considers the point in compounding or preparation of the product as it relates to raw material processing, final product processing, or something in between these two points.

Statutes and regulations provide the definitions to enable characterization of a particular product. The definitions are too lengthy for reproduction in this text; however, the following will provide the essential components of the definitions to help distinguish between the products encountered most often in the health care industry.

DRUG: Articles intended for use in the diagnosis, cure, mitigation, treatment, or prevention of disease in man or other animals; articles intended to affect the structure or any function of the body of man or other animals. Does not include devices [9].

DEVICE: An instrument, apparatus, implement, machine, contrivance, implant, *in vitro* reagent, or other similar or related article intended for use in the diagnosis of disease or other conditions, or in the cure, mitigation, treatment, or prevention of disease, in man or other animals, or intended to affect the structure or any function of the body of man or other animals. A device does not achieve any of its principal intended purposes through chemical action within or on the body and is not dependent upon being metabolized for the achievement of any of its principal intended purposes [10].

BIOLOGICAL PRODUCT: Any virus, therapeutic serum, toxin, antitoxin, vaccine, blood, blood component or derivative, allergenic product, or analogous product, or arsphenamine or its derivatives (or any other trivalent organic arsenic compound) [11]. These categories are further clarified by regulation [12].

The drug and device definitions share some of the same components. Both drugs and devices are *intended for use in the diagnosis, cure, mitigation, treatment, or prevention of disease in man or other animals*. Both drugs and devices are *intended to affect the structure or function of the body of man or other animals*. There are, however, distinctions to be made between drugs and devices through their definitions. Drugs are characterized as articles which are *not* devices. Devices are characterized as *an instrument, apparatus, implement, machine, contrivance, implant, or* in vitro *reagent*. In contrast to a drug, a device *does not achieve any of its principal intended purposes through chemical action* and *is not dependent upon being metabolized for the achievement of any of its principal intended purposes*. Thus, drugs and devices are mutually exclusive in that a drug cannot be a device and a device cannot be a drug.

A biologic, however, may also be a drug or a device and therefore may be subject to additional controls. To illustrate, consider the development of two proteins: one an endogenous blood component produced either by separation from blood sources or prepared synthetically; the other an exogenous substance structurally not similar to a known human blood component yet functionally active in a way a known blood component might work. Most likely, the endogenous protein would be considered a biologic and subject to both drug and biologic regulations. The exogenous substance most likely would not be considered a biologic and thus would be subject only to drug regulations. Careful consideration must be given when faced with this type of situation. Early discussions with the FDA are recommended to help avoid surprises later in how the product will be handled by the FDA.

9.7   Functions of regulatory affairs

The functions of regulatory affairs can be divided into four categories:
1. Submissions,
2. Compliance,
3. Enforcement, and
4. Miscellaneous.

Keep in mind as you read through this section the concept of integration and the broad perspective needed by regulatory affairs for their role in linking the various aspects of product development and marketing.

9.7.1   Submissions

Before a product can be tested or marketed, an application sometimes must be filed with the FDA. When a product is a new drug [13], meaning it is not generally recognized as safe and effective and is not grandfathered, a New Drug Application (NDA) must be submitted to the FDA prior to marketing. "Generally recognized" means that more than just one or a few people agree or disagree as to the product's safety and efficacy. Whether a product is "grandfathered" is a term used to describe the process by which the law provides an exception to the rule requiring prior FDA approval for some products to be marketed.

Devices are categorized into three classifications, designated Class I, II, or III [14]. Prior to marketing a Class I or II device, a Premarket Notification must be sent to the FDA ninety days prior to introducing the product into interstate commerce for commercial sale [15]. A Class III device is one which requires prior approval of the FDA before commercial marketing may begin [16].

Submissions requirements for biological products are governed by the PHS Act [17]. Products of this type require two different submissions: one for the purpose of describing the product, called a Product License Application (PLA); and the second for the purpose of describing the facilities used to manufacture the product, referred to as an Establishment License Application (ELA) [18].

Affecting the type of submission required by FDA is the "stage of development" spoken of earlier. The three stages are:

1. Investigational (learning phase),
2. Marketing (routine operations), and
3. Post-marketing (improvements).

By categorizing a product within one of these stages, issues are narrowed and brought into focus, providing a means by which one can develop an organized time-line for completing required tasks.

Remember that the FDA is a stranger to a new product. Telling a story—beginning to end—for the purpose of educating the FDA reviewer is of paramount importance to help streamline the review process and hopefully eliminate delays from reviewer questions. This beginning-to-end story is also helpful if a review of the FDA's decision becomes necessary. Only the information contained in the administrative record will be considered. Thus, failure to provide the necessary underlying foundation for the product claims being made surely will affect the outcome of any challenge to an FDA order.

At the investigational stage, there are two types of product submissions to be considered depending on the character of the product. Drugs and biologics may require the submission of a Notice of Claimed Exemption for a New Drug (IND) [19]. A device may require submission of an Investigational Device Exemption (IDE) [20].

Submissions at the marketing stage differ in terminology depending on whether the product is a drug, device, or biologic. The content of each submission, however, is basically the same—to provide a complete story about the product from beginning to end to educate the reviewer and create a complete and comprehensible administrative record. Drugs generally require either a NDA or Abbreviated NDA [21]. Devices require either a Premarket Notification [510(k)] [22] or a Premarket Approval Application (PMA) [23]. Biologics require submission of both a PLA and an ELA [24].

Post-marketing submissions cover a broad range of topics, including such things as:

1. Establishment registration [25],
2. Product listing [26],
3. Adverse reaction reporting [27],
4. Supplemental applications,
5. Periodic reports, and
6. Advertising and promotional copy.

Many of these topics are addressed in various places throughout the laws and regulations already cited for the different product types.

One last type of submission to be considered is a document called a "master file." This document can be prepared and submitted to any FDA center reviewing a product. Its purpose is to provide information to the FDA on a particular product, process, facility, or procedure that would apply to many products under review by that center of FDA or that may be used where the sponsor of the product wants to allow another company to reference the information but wants to protect the confidentiality of the information.

In summary, the submissions aspect of regulatory affairs is to bring together and integrate the technical and marketing data for a product and advocate for the product in a persuasive, complete, and balanced presentation.

9.7.2 Compliance

Compliance is an area of regulatory affairs that has many facets. Three of these facets deal with the "good practice" regulations. The remaining three facets focus on reviews of study data, established policies and procedures, and commitments made in regulatory or other submissions.

9.7.2.1 Good laboratory practice (GLP)

The first of the good practice regulations are those that deal with GLP for conducting nonclinical laboratory studies [28]. Of particular importance is the scope of applicability of these regulations, which establishes the studies that are affected by and that must be conducted in accordance with these regulations.

A nonclinical laboratory study is an *in vivo* or *in vitro* experiment in which a test article is studied prospectively under laboratory conditions to determine its *safety*. A nonclinical laboratory study does not include basic exploratory studies carried out to determine whether a test article has any potential utility or to determine physical or chemical characteristics of a test article. This would include such tests as identity, strength, quality, and purity as opposed to safety or efficacy. Thus, unnecessary application of these regulations is burdensome in that a study can become very costly and overly time consuming. This was not the goal of these regulations.

Another important definition is that of the "test facility." This is defined as a person who actually conducts a nonclinical laboratory study (i.e., actually uses the test article in a test system). Thus, a sample analysis lab is not, by definition, covered by this regulation. However, in keeping with the concept that the regulations were developed to prevent data mix-ups or falsification, it is prudent to consider having adequate procedures and documentation in place for all laboratory work.

9.7.2.2 Good manufacturing practice (GMP)

There are three regulations that deal with manufacturing: one for drugs [29], another for medical devices [30], and yet another for blood and blood components [31]. Here again, proper characterization of the product is essential to determine the appropriate regulations with which one must comply.

When dealing with drug products, the stage of manufacture determines whether the GMP regulations or some other criteria apply. Drug manufacture can be divided into three steps: preparation of the (1) drug substance, (2) bulk drug product, and (3) finished pharmaceutical. The GMP regulations technically apply only to categories (2) and (3), bulk drug product and finished pharmaceuticals, respectively. Preparation of the drug substance (otherwise known as a bulk pharmaceutical chemical) is dealt with in a guideline entitled "Guide to Inspection of Bulk Pharmaceutical Chemical Manufacturing." The guideline, though not having the force of a regulation, emphasizes the same approach as the GMP regulations but also accounts for the need for allowances to be made when dealing with various types of processes such as fermentation, extraction, or chemical syntheses and/or reactions.

To complicate things further, stage of development determines applicability of regulations or guidelines. For instance, clinical product manufacture is addressed in a guideline entitled "Preparation of Investigational New Drug Products."

Sometimes, regulations are proposed by the FDA yet never finalized. They nevertheless remain useful for guidance. A good example of such a case is the set of regulations proposed in 1976 entitled "Current Good Manufacturing Practice in the Manufacture, Processing, Packing, or Holding of Large Volume Parenterals for Human Use." Though these regulations were never finalized by FDA, the concepts of aseptic processing contained therein provide a very helpful starting point when dealing with aseptic processing. As part of a change in the regulatory environment, government has been emphasizing voluntary compliance over rulemaking; thus, many proposed or tentative regulations have not yet come to fruition.

9.7.2.3 Good clinical practice (GCP)
The third area of good practice concepts relates to clinical investigations. Though there is no regulation specifically entitled "Good Clinical Practice," there are several regulations nonetheless which govern the conduct of clinical studies.

To protect individuals participating in a clinical study, by regulation each participant must receive information about the study and product/compound they are about to receive as part of the study so that they can make an informed decision whether or not to participate in the study. FDA regulations entitled "Protection of Human Subjects" [32] set forth the requirements for informed consent.

As a means of independent monitoring to protect the rights and welfare of clinical subjects, the FDA requires that studies be conducted under the continuing review of a committee independent of the study sponsor called an Institutional Review Board (IRB) [33]. The regulations are quite specific as to the organization and personnel who make up this board. These regulations also specify board functions and operation, as well as the records and reports that are to be kept. One function of the IRB is to review the information to be provided a clinical subject upon which their informed consent will be obtained.

The FDA has promulgated regulations that provide guidance to sponsors and clinical investigators. The IND regulations have a section which discusses the responsibilities of sponsors and investigators [34]. The IDE regulations similarly address the subject [20].

The FDA expects on-going review of clinical investigations. To provide assistance in this area, the agency has issued a guideline entitled "Guideline for the Monitoring of Clinical Investigations," which explains what monitoring is needed and how to properly document the monitoring.

9.7.2.4 Study/data audits
This area of regulatory compliance focuses on the review of raw data contained in reports. In the case of good laboratory or good clinical practices, it means assuring the data contained in written study reports matches the raw data obtained during the study. In manufacturing, it means assuring the raw data in the batch record is consistent with the written product specifications.

9.7.2.5 Corporate policies and procedures

The good practice regulations represent only the minimum standards expected to be maintained. In most instances, companies will impose stricter standards on themselves than are required by the FDA, since they must consider product liability and the negative effect a mistake could have on the public relations and financial affairs of the company. The FDA also will look to see if these self-imposed procedures are followed, since a failure to do so at this level suggests the potential for failure in following good practice regulations. Thus, audits should include a review of policies and procedures implemented by the company, as well as good practice-required procedures.

9.7.2.6 Submissions commitments

As a final regulatory compliance check, there should be periodic reviews of submissions made to the FDA and other entities, whether governmental or business partners, to assure that representations made to these parties is an accurate reflection of current policies, procedures, and practices. There is great potential in this area for mistakes when working with off-site locations for manufacture or for companies that market internationally and have made representations to various foreign governments. Rarely do any two countries have identical requirements for testing, manufacture, or marketing.

9.7.2.7 Summary

The underlying concept of compliance is communication—through written policies, procedures, and other such documents. It is through this written communication that the people throughout the company involved with the product are integrated in such a way as to assure the end product is in fact what it is expected to be, each and every time. Anytime there is a deviation from the plan, there is the very real possibility the end result will be different than expected. Unfortunately, technology is not always sufficiently advanced to be able to distinguish subtle yet sometimes harmful differences.

9.7.3 Enforcement

Enforcement is the end result of a lack of integration. It implies a failure in the systems designed to prevent mistakes and inadvertent or untested changes. There are two methods of enforcement: imposition of civil or criminal penalties, and product liability suits.

   Civil remedies available to the FDA include such things as seizure and detention of product wherein the specific suspect product is held from distribution. Another remedy is injunctive relief wherein, by court order, there is a prohibition against further distribution. Failure to comply with these remedies permits a court to find an individual in contempt of court and subject to fines and/or imprisonment.

   Criminal penalties can result from gross or repeated failure to meet FDA requirements. The privilege of doing business carries with it the burden of responsibility to protect the public welfare. There is, unfortunately, a very real temptation by some to short-cut the safeguards imposed by the FDA and the laws it enforces.

   Although case law suggests [35] it is the Chief Executive Officer (CEO) who will be held responsible, the more technologically sophisticated the compliance requirements become, the less likely it is to realistically hold only the CEO responsible for compliance. Thus, the technologically trained managers may soon find the burden of responsibility shifting their way. Irrespective of the above, any individual found to have presented false data to the FDA is subject to criminal penalties.

More real and surely more damaging, however, are product liability suits. These are costly to defend and carry the potential for very large damage awards. There are several legal theories upon which a product liability suit may be brought. They include express warranty, negligent misrepresentation, negligent manufacture, design defect, strict liability, implied warranty, and fraud or knowing misrepresentation.

Express warranty, negligent misrepresentation, and fraud problems usually result from claims made in labeling or advertisements. Implied warranties of merchantability or fitness for a particular use have their basis in the Uniform Commercial Code, which deals with the sale of goods to consumers.

Design defects relate to a problem of foreseeability of danger in the end use of a product by a reasonable, prudent person. Foreseeable misuse must be considered in the design of a product. Another, more specific, example of a design defect would be the difference between using an aseptic manufacturing process rather than an equally viable terminal sterilization process. The terminal sterilization process provides far more assurance of sterility as compared to an aseptic manufacturing process. All else being equal, the less risky alternative should be the method of choice.

Strict liability basically means that for some products considered to be inherently dangerous, if there is an injury, liability will automatically attach.

The theory of negligent manufacture has a special pitfall—something called negligence *per se*. Negligence has two components: negligent conduct and negligent liability. "Negligent conduct" merely means acting in a careless way. "Negligent liability" attaches when negligent conduct results in an injury. There are four parts to negligent liability: the existence of a duty owed to another, a breach of that duty, injury caused by the negligent conduct, and actual injury or damages. The marketing of products, particularly products in the health care industry, carries with it various duties to the individuals who use the product. So, the threshold question is whether or not one of the duties has been breached. One way to establish a breach is to look to the industry standards of operation and assess whether there has been a significant short-fall in performance. If so, negligent conduct exists and all that remains to be shown is that there was in fact an injury and that it was caused by the negligent conduct. Generally, the evidence required to show a breach is difficult to establish. The concept of negligence *per se,* however, works to lessen the plaintiff's burden in establishing a breach. All that is required to establish a breach, and thus negligent conduct, is a showing that there has been a violation of a statute (e.g., an FDA regulation). Compliance, therefore, or the lack of it, can carry a heavy burden of responsibility.

9.7.4 Miscellaneous

There are a few other items to be briefly mentioned. Consideration and investigation should be undertaken to determine any state requirements with which compliance is needed. California is one state that has facility and product registration requirements [36]. In some circumstances, the California State Board of Pharmacy requires that a licensed pharmacist be responsible for manufacturing [37].

Both state and federal laws address the manufacture and handling of controlled substances (e.g., habit-forming drugs) [38].

Lastly, there are provisions for the FDA to provide certain development and marketing incentives for sponsors of orphan products (e.g., those products having little market as a result of the few number of individuals afflicted with a particular condition but who nevertheless need the product) [39].

9.8 Conclusion

The regulatory process is an interactive process that cannot and should not be rushed. It is highly dependent on the quality of communication between people operating under a structure of rules and regulations often intentionally left vague to provide flexibility and promote dialogue.

Defining and keeping focused on the relevant issues eliminates unnecessary work. The key to achieving this is through proper characterization of the product classification, stage of development, and stage of manufacture.

Skills that promote success in working with the regulators include knowing the rules that define their structure, a strong ability to communicate both verbally and in writing, organization, and a penchant for detail and documentation.

References

[1]   21 USC

[2]   42 USC

[3]   5 USC 551

[4]   21 CFR 10.90

[5]   United States Pharmacopeia/National Formulary Constitution

[6]   "USPC Communications Policy," *USP XXII/NF XVII*

[7]   FDA Compliance Policy Guide No. 7132.05, 1 Oct. 1980

[8]   21 USC 351 and 352, et seq.

[9]   FDC Act § 201(g)(1)

[10] FDC Act § 201(h)

[11] Virus, Serum, and Toxin Act of 1944

[12] 21 CFR 600.3(h)

[13] FDC Act § 505

[14] FDC Act § 513

[15] FDC Act § 510(k)

[16] FDC Act § 515

[17] 351 Public Health Service Act

[18] 21 CFR 601

[19] 21 CFR 312

[20] 21 CFR 812 and 813

[21] 21 CFR 314

[22] FDC Act § 510

[23] FDC Act § 515

[24] 21 CFR 601

[25] 21 CFR 207, 607, 807

[26] 21 CFR 207, 607, 807

[27]   21 CFR 314, 606, 803
[28]   21 CFR 58
[29]   21 CFR 211
[30]   21 CFR 820
[31]   21 CFR 606
[32]   21 CFR 50
[33]   21 CFR 56
[34]   21 CFR 312, Subpart D
[35]   U.S. v. Park (U.S. Sup. Ct. 1975) 421 U.S. 658, 95 S. Ct. 1903
[36]   Health and Safety Code § 26685
[37]   Business and Professions Code § 4050
[38]   21 CFR 1300
[39]   FDC Act § 515, et seq.

10 Regulatory issues—Europe

R. Wikberg-Leonardi and D. Mulder

Content

10.1 Europe is not only EC

The plans for changing the regulatory process in Europe in preparation for the 1993 "one market" Europe are still under discussion. The outline is that there will be a central Medicines Agency with whom all high-tech products will be filed. After review of the dossier by this central Medicines Agency, there is going to be a binding agreement that all member states will have to accept.

For conventional products, the planned system is that the dossier is submitted to one country (of sponsor's choice). After approval in the country where the dossier was originally submitted, other member states will mutually recognize the registration of the drug. Only if there are differences of opinion between the member states will the dossier for a conventional product be referred to the central agency.

Europe is the second-smallest (after Australia) of the seven continents of the world. In size, it accounts for less than 6.6% of the world's total land area. However, because of its location, considerable economic resources, and population (about 685 million or 13.2% of the world's total in 1989), this small continent has played and continues to play a major role in world affairs.

In political and economic discussions, Europe is defined as the area lying west of the former Soviet Union and Turkey. The countries of Europe are listed below with their estimated populations (1990 World Almanac and Book of Facts, 1989).

Country	Area (sq. mi)	Population (1989 est.)	Capitol
Albania	11,100	3,201,000	Tirana
Andorra	185	56,000	Andorra la Vella
Austria	32,374	7,500,000	Vienna
Belgium	11,779	9,897,000	Brussels
Bulgaria	44,365	9,037,000	Sofia
Cyprus	3,572	696,000	Nicosia
Czechoslovakia[1]	49,365	15,661,000	Prague
Denmark	16,663	5,074,000	Copenhagen
Finland	130,119	4,990,000	Helsinki
France	220,668	55,813,000	Paris
Germany[1]	137,743	76,898,000	Berlin
Gibraltar	2.5	29,048	—
Greece	51,146	10,048,000	Athens
Hungary	35,919	10,571,000	Budapest
Iceland	39,769	251,000	Reykjavik
Irish Republic	27,137	3,734,000	Dublin
Italy	116,303	57,439,000	Rome
Liechtenstein	62	30,000	Vaduz
Luxembourg	998	369,000	Luxembourg
Malta	122	358,000	Valletta

[1] Since this chapter was written and finalized, and at the time of publication, the European map has changed.

Country	Area (sq. mi)	Population (1989 est.)	Capitol
Monaco	.06	29,000	Monaco
Netherlands	15,770	14,689,000	Amsterdam
Norway	125,181	4,204,000	Oslo
Poland	120,727	38,389,000	Warsaw
Portugal	36,390	10,240,000	Lisbon
Romania	91,699	23,155,000	Bucharest
San Marino	24	23,000	San Marino
Spain	194,896	39,784,000	Madrid
Sweden	173,731	8,371,000	Stockholm
Switzerland	15,941	6,485,000	Bern
Turkey	301,381	55,377,000	Ankara
United Kingdom	94,226	56,648,000	London
U.S.S.R. (former)[1]	8,649,496	287,015,000	Moscow
Vatican City	108.7	750	—
Yugoslavia[1]	1 98,766	23,753,000	Belgrade

Owing to its political fragmentation, Europe has always recorded the highest volume of international trade of any region in the world. Inevitably, as the interdependence of countries has increased in the wake of such economic groupings as the European Economic Community (EC), European Free Trade Association (EFTA), and Council for Mutual Economic Aid (COMECON), and as the continent's standard of living has risen, figures that were already high have become even higher. About two-thirds of all commerce between countries has its origin or destination in a European state, and about 40% of the world's total trade is carried on by the EC nations. Moreover, about three-fourths of all of Europe's trade is with other European countries, and about one-third of all American trade is carried on with Europe. Europe's major trading nation is Germany, followed by the United Kingdom, France, and Italy.

In the review of regulatory issues, an overview of requirements of the western European countries will be given. The countries that belong to COMECON will not be part of this review.

10.1.1 EC

The EC was established by treaty in 1957. The original members—Belgium, Germany, France, Italy, Luxembourg, and the Netherlands—formulated a treaty with the common aim of an even closer union of the people of Europe. The membership has now risen to twelve with the addition of the United Kingdom, Denmark, Ireland, Greece, Spain, and Portugal. The community's aim is to integrate their economies, coordinate social developments, and bring about political union of the democratic states of Europe. At the time of this printing, the members had agreed that a single European market which would remove all barriers to free trade and free movement of capital, services, goods, and people would take effect at the end of 1992.

An EC "directive" is an instrument that provides a framework for national legislation. The directive sets out all the principles and criteria for the regulation of a particular area but does not have to be translated exactly into national laws. When national legislation and an EC directive are at variance, the EC directive takes precedence.

The objective of the EC directives on pharmaceuticals is to achieve the harmonization of laws, regulations, and administrative provisions relating to the placing on the market of medicinal products (as defined in articles 1.1 and 1.2 of Directive 65/65/EC). The criteria on which a marketing approval is assessed are safety, quality, efficacy, and economic impact. These criteria and their interpretation and evolution have been progressively harmonized within Europe so that, insofar as is practicable within the constraints of medical practice, the granting of a marketing authorization in each member state is conducted on a similar basis and in a comparable way.

As EC legislation on pharmaceuticals has evolved, the increasing level of harmonization under the directives should make it easier for national licensing authorities to recognize each other's decisions. EC directives have been promulgated to further this process (Directive 75/319/EC and Directive 87/22/EC) by setting up the Committee for Proprietary Medicinal Products (CPMP) Multi-State Application procedure and the "Bio/High-tech Concertation" procedure.

The CPMP, a committee of representatives of the national registration authorities, was established in accordance with Directive 75/319/EC in 1976. Under the aegis of this committee, a procedure to enable rapid mutual recognition of a licensing authorization granted by one member state to some or all of the other member states was established.
Developments in the area of biotechnology have resulted in a new range of pharmaceutical products, in relation to which all member states are facing new problems of evaluation. The EC has, therefore, established under Directive 87/22/EC a mechanism whereby the CPMP will consider applications for new products of biotechnology prior to their evaluation and granting of a marketing authorization by a member state. This "Bio/High-tech Concertation" procedure has given greater harmonization of decision processes within the EC.

10.1.2 EFTA

The EFTA consists of Austria, Iceland, Norway, Sweden, Switzerland, and associated member Finland. It was created on 4 January 1960 to gradually reduce customs duties and quantitative restrictions between members on industrial products. Compared to the EC organization, there is no strong coordination of pharmaceutical legislation within the EFTA group. Within the Nordic countries— Denmark, Iceland, Norway, Sweden, and Finland—there are guidelines to prepare applications for submission of drugs. The same file can be submitted to all five Nordic countries. Denmark, besides being a Nordic country, also is a member of the EC and, therefore, is included in the EC procedure. Austria and Switzerland have their own rules for registration of pharmaceuticals, but an EC file includes all information necessary and can be submitted both to Austria and Switzerland.

10.2 Issues in the EC

10.2.1 Alternate procedures for registration

Since 1977, alternate procedures have been available for obtaining authorization to market medicinal products within the member states of the EC. Instead of submitting separate applications to the regulatory authorities of the individual member states (termed "competent authorities"), a common application to five or more member states could be submitted after first having obtained a marketing authorization in one member state. When Directive 83/570/EC became effective in November 1985, major changes were made to the EC procedure. The minimum number of member states to which a common application had to be made was reduced from five to two, and the member states to which the application is addressed were instructed to take the authorization granted by the first member state into due consideration.

This procedure is generally called the "Multi-State" procedure. It can be used for new drug applications, as well as for abridged applications (generics). This procedure is not compulsory, however. Applications also can be submitted under purely national procedures.

Directive 87/22/EC, which came into effect on 1 July 1987, created a special EC procedure for the coordination of national decisions relating to the marketing of high technology medicinal products, in particular those derived from biotechnology. The use of this so-called "concertation" procedure is mandatory for the majority of products for both human and veterinary use that are derived from biotechnology.

Thus, there are currently three procedures that can be used for obtaining marketing approval in the EC member states:

1. Multi-state,
2. National, and
3. Concertation.

In addition to the procedures for applying for marketing authorization, Article 11 of Directive 75/319/EC, as amended by Directive 83/570/EC, enables a member state or the Commission of the EC to refer to the CPMP, for an opinion, cases where a proprietary medicinal product has been authorized for use in one or more member states and refused authorization, suspended, or withdrawn from the market in others. The opinion of the CPMP, which must be given within 60 days, will concern only the grounds on which authorization has been suspended, refused, or withdrawn.

The rules governing proprietary medicinal products for human use have, to a large extent, been harmonized within the member states of the EC. These rules, which apply equally to applications submitted through national procedures and to applications submitted through EC procedures, are contained in a series of legal texts: the directives.

A "Notice to Applicants" has been prepared to facilitate the compilation of the dossier as required by the directives. It specifies the data and documents which must accompany the application for a marketing authorization and describes the standard format for the presentation of dossiers and expert reports. The notice to applicants presents the harmonized view of the member states on how the legal requirements may be met. It has no legal status and in case of doubt, reference should be made to the relevant EC directives.

In addition, working parties of the CPMP have prepared and continue to prepare guidelines on the conduct of tests and clinical trials of proprietary medicinal products. These guidelines are intended to give detailed but flexible advice for manufacturers. Guidelines are not binding to the manufactures; however, deviations from the guidelines must be justified in the dossier.

The above-mentioned texts have been brought together in a single collection of five volumes; the bibliographical references are given in section 10.4. When necessary, each volume is updated to reflect the current EC legislation.

The expected installation in 1993 of a single market without borders implies that pharmaceuticals authorized in one member state will be able to circulate freely throughout the Community. Experience gained with the CPMP procedures has highlighted difficulties in accepting the principles of mutual recognition of marketing authorizations by the twelve national authorities.

The Commission of the EC has forwarded proposals on the future "post-1992" system for the authorization of the marketing of pharmaceuticals in the EC. The new proposals provide for a three-tier system:

1. A decentralized system for most drug products, whereby approval in one state would be recognized by other states;
2. A strengthened CPMP as a central body, with strong scientific back-up and binding opinions, mandatory for biotechnology products and optional for new chemical entities; also for other products for which one state disputes approval by another state under the decentralized procedure; and
3. National procedures for drug applications limited to a single member state (only possible during a transitional stage).

10.2.2 Concertation procedure

10.2.2.1 Purpose and scope

The objective of the concertation procedure is to resolve issues at the EC level within the CPMP before a national decision is reached concerning the marketing of a new medicinal product. These questions would pertain to the quality, safety, and efficacy of pharmaceuticals developed by means of biotechnology processes or other high technology procedures.

This procedure is obligatory for all pharmaceuticals developed by means of the following biotechnological processes:

1. Recombinant DNA technology;
2. Controlled expression of genes coding for biologically active proteins in prokaryotes and eukaryotes, including transformed mammalian cells; and
3. Hybridoma and monoclonal antibody methods.

Applications for marketing biotechnology medicinal products do not have to be referred to the CPMP if the applicant certifies that application for marketing authorization is being made to only one member state, that no other application for the product has been made to the authorities of another member state during the preceding five years, and that authorization will not be sought in any other member state for five years. Should an application for authorization subsequently be made to another member state within the five-year period, it will automatically be referred to the CPMP by the second member state.

In addition, applicants for marketing authorization for the following groups of products may request the authorities of a member state to refer the matter to the CPMP for consideration before any national decision on the application is reached:

1. Medicinal products developed by other biotechnological processes which constitute a significant innovation;
2. Medicinal products administered by means of new delivery systems which constitute a significant innovation;
3. Medicinal products containing a new substance or having an entirely new indication which is of significant therapeutic interest;
4. New medicinal products based on radio-isotopes which are of significant therapeutic interest; and
5. Medicinal products the manufacture of which employs processes which demonstrate a significant technical advance, such as two-dimensional electrophoresis under micro-gravity.

If the national authorities are satisfied that the medicinal product has the significant innovatory character claimed, they shall refer the application to the CPMP. The CPMP will consider the question of innovation and decide whether it is competent to consider the application.

10.2.2.2   Submission and timetable of the application

The timetable for the concertation procedure is set by filing the application in the first member state. When this member state accepts it as a valid application, the member state becomes the "rapporteur" of the concertation procedure. The applicant notifies the CPMP of the application.

The applicant should immediately (within two to three weeks) submit a formal application with a full dossier to those other member states in which authorization is being sought. The application does not have to be submitted to all member states of the EC. To facilitate applications, all member states have agreed that the receipt of a full dossier in English is satisfactory for the purposes of starting the procedure, provided translations of appropriate parts are supplied within 30 days. A full dossier plus a summary is supplied to the CPMP Secretariat. A summary of the dossier, consisting of at least the administrative information, the "Summary of the Product Characteristics", and the expert reports and tabulated formats (or equivalent documents in the case of products not yet covered by the EC directives) must be sent to those member states not directly concerned by the application.

The rapporteur member state initiates the concertation procedure when all of the member states concerned have received the file. Up to ten working days may elapse between receipt of the dossier and commencement of the procedure to allow the member states to validate the dossier. The concertation timetable will be circulated to all member states, and the secretariat of the CPMP by the rapporteur and the applicant will be notified.

Examination of the application by the CPMP takes place at the same time as examination of the application by the authorities of the rapporteur member state. In case of concertation applications, no previous assessment by a national authority will have been prepared. Therefore, bio/high technology applications are likely to be treated as exceptional by the CPMP. The normal review period of 120 days is thus usually extended by 90 days. These time limits may be expanded where the applicant is required to provide additional information, orally or in writing. For its part, the CPMP is required to complete its consideration 30 days before the expiration of these time limits so that the national authorities have time to consider the opinion of the CPMP before reaching a final decision. To this end, the CPMP and the applicant are kept informed of any decision by the rapporteur to extend the time limit or to stop the clock by requesting additional information from the company.

The rapporteur member state prepares an evaluation report with questions and circulates it to all member states and the CPMP secretariat; the questions are sent to the applicant company within 45 days of the commencement of the procedure, and the clock is stopped. Within the next 60 days, all member states are invited to add comments and questions to the evaluation report of the rapporteur. The rapporteur prepares a compilation of all the objections, and these are discussed by the CPMP. Within the next 45 days, the final list of objections is forwarded to the applicant company.

The company then sends to all member states a consolidated response to the questions within a period negotiated with the rapporteur (usually within three months). Subsequently, the rapporteur starts the clock again. Thirty days after restarting the clock, all member states involved inform the rapporteur and CPMP of their conclusion on the company's response. The rapporteur then sets a date for obtaining the opinion of the CPMP that must be 30 days before the expiration of the overall time limit.

If the company wishes a hearing, this should be confirmed by the company to the rapporteur and the secretariat 30 working days in advance of the scheduled CPMP meeting date. Applicants should discuss the content of written documents to be used in conjunction with a hearing with the rapporteur.

The opinion of the CPMP will be concerned exclusively with the quality, safety, and efficacy of the product. The opinion, which is not binding, will be transmitted to the applicant and to the member states. The member states concerned by the application are required to reach a decision on the action they intend to take following the CPMP's opinion within 30 days of its receipt. Those member states originally not involved will consider the opinion of the CPMP when examining any subsequent application for authorization in respect of the same product.

10.2.3 Preparation of the application

As far as possible, applicants should follow the guidelines for preparing dossiers and expert reports as given in the Notice to Applicants. However, these guidelines may not be entirely appropriate in all cases.

It is advisable to discuss the preparation of a dossier with the national authority of the rapporteur member state at an early stage. In general, a dossier consists of the following parts:

Part I Summary of the Dossier
- A. Administrative data, including an index for all documentation submitted
- B. Summary of Product Characteristics
- C. Expert reports on chemical, toxicological and clinical documentation

Part II Chemical, Pharmaceutical and Biological Documentation
- A. Composition
- B. Method of preparation
- C. Control of starting materials
- D. Control tests on intermediate products
- E. Control tests on the finished product
- F. Stability

Part III Toxicological and Pharmacological Documentation
- A. Single dose toxicity
- B. Repeated dose toxicity
- C. Reproduction studies
- D. Mutagenic potential
- E. Oncogenic/carcinogenic potential
- F. Pharmacodynamics
- G. Pharmacokinetics
- H. Local tolerance
- I. Other information

Part IV Clinical documentation
- A. Clinical pharmacology
- B. Clinical experience

   C.   Other information
Part V   Special particulars
   A.   Dosage form
   B.   Samples
   C.   Manufacturers authorization(s)
   D.   Marketing authorization(s)

In the twelve EC member states, nine official languages are spoken: English, French, Dutch, Italian, Spanish, Portuguese, Danish, Greek, and German. Although most countries prefer applications drafted in the national language, all countries except Spain accept submission of Parts II, III, and IV of the application in English. Some countries require Part I to be written in the national language, all countries require a translation of the package insert and the labelling. The number of copies of the application to be submitted to the authorities of each member state varies per country and is listed in the Notice to Applicants.

Some EC member states require the submission of samples of the pharmaceutical product as it will be marketed simultaneously with the submission of the application . Other member states should not be sent samples with an application for an authorization unless requested by the authorities. Moreover, samples of the active ingredients must be supplied as a matter of course in some member states. Details are provided in the Notice to Applicants.

10.2.4 Expert reports

In accordance with Directive 75/319/EC, the chemical-pharmaceutical, pharmaco-toxicological, and clinical parts of the dossier should each include an expert report. An expert report should not just summarize the data but should include a critical evaluation of the properties of the product, discussing deviations from the guidelines and the Notice the Applicants. Great care should be taken in the preparation of the expert reports, as well-prepared reports are essential for efficient and effective review of applications by the authorities. Failure to provide properly prepared expert reports constitutes grounds for refusing the application.

Suitably qualified and experienced persons must be used to compile these reports. Their nationalities are not relevant. The expert is expected to take and defend a clear position on the product in the light of current scientific knowledge. The expert need not have been personally involved in the performance of the tests and need not even be employed by the company. Instead, the task can be delegated to a recognized expert from outside. When selecting an expert, it is important to realize that the expert would usually be expected to represent the company if an oral hearing is to be held.

In the Notice to Applicants, the general qualifications and experience recommended for the three experts are defined, as is the format of the expert report. An expert report should bear the signature of the expert and the place and date of its issue. A brief curriculum vitae of the expert should be attached to the report and the expert's professional relationship to the applicant stated.

The expert reports must be preceded by a "product profile" of the application as an introduction to the report. The product profile consists of one to two pages; it is a brief extract of the summary of product characteristics and repeats the type of application, the chemical and pharmacokinetic properties, the indications, the precautions, marketing authorizations already granted, and the post-marketing surveillance program.

10.2.5 The role of the rapporteur

The first member state to which an application is submitted acts as the rapporteur. The applicant should initiate direct contact with the authority of the rapporteur in a very early stage of dossier preparation. Only after this consultation should a complete application for marketing authorization be submitted to the authorities of the EC member states, including the rapporteur member state. The rapporteur will refer the application to the CPMP in accordance with the special concertation procedure. The role of the rapporteur includes determination of the timetable, as well as close liaison with the applicant and other member states concerned. The rapporteur prepares the initial assessment report, compiles the objections of all member states, and reports at the CPMP meeting on the resolution of objections. The rapporteur is, in practice, the link between the company and the CPMP.

The company must take great care in fully cooperating with the rapporteur and should not hesitate to ask the rapporteur for advice. The rapporteur should be consulted before any documentation is sent to the CPMP members and should be fully informed of the company's proposed time schedule for submitting responses to objections raised by the CPMP.

10.2.6 Review process

The rapporteur determines the start of the clock of the concertation procedure. Before the procedure starts, all member states should have received the dossier/summary.

The rapporteur prepares an assessment report with questions which is circulated to all member states, who are then invited to add comments and questions. In practice, the evaluation of a CPMP dossier by the national authorities is not different from evaluation of a national application, with the exception of the time-frame for completing the process.

Where applicable, experts from outside the government offices are invited to review parts of the dossier. At the CPMP meeting, all objections are discussed, and a consolidated list of objections is prepared and forwarded to the company.

An applicant company may provide the CPMP with a written response and/or may request a hearing to present the responses orally. Applicants should bear in mind that oral or written explanations are made to the CPMP as a whole (i.e., to the representatives from all EC member states). Although the authorities not directly concerned by the application will not necessarily have seen the complete dossier, they will have seen the summaries of the dossier, the objections of the member states to which the application was submitted, and any available assessment reports.

The pharmaceutical part of a dossier on a biotechnological product is assessed in the CPMP Ad Hoc Working Party on Biotechnology/Pharmacy. Preclinical and clinical issues are discussed at the CPMP meeting. The opinion of the working party is usually adopted by the CPMP. The opinion of the CPMP is exclusively based on the comments and objections put forward by the member states concerned. Issues not raised previously in writing by the individual Member States are not discussed at the CPMP meeting. The opinion of the CPMP or, in the case of divergent opinions, the opinions of its members are immediately forwarded to the applicant and to the member states.

The opinion of the CPMP is not binding and does not replace national decisions. However, within 30 days of the receipt of the opinion, member states involved in the application must decide what action to take based on the committee's opinion and notify the CPMP of that decision. The member states keep the CPMP informed of the actions they are taking until such time as a definitive decision is adopted on a national level.

10.2.7 Labeling

The requirements for labels and package inserts have not yet been harmonized in the EC, although the directive on package inserts and labeling has been published. Member states should comply with this directive before January 1, 1993; from January 1993 onward, applications which do not contain labeling and package inserts in compliance with the directive will be refused.

It is advisable to include proposals for labels and package inserts in the language of each country and in accord with the national legal requirements in the dossier. The national legal requirements vary widely between the member states, ranging from no requirements at all to texts dictated word-for-word by the authorities. In all cases, package inserts are based on Section IB of the dossier, the Summary of Product Characteristics.

Some of the EC member states require two package inserts for a product—one directed at the treating physician and one at the patient. The proposed label and package inserts are generally only reviewed at the final stage of the registration process (i.e., after the documentation on the safety, efficacy, and quality of the product have been approved).

10.2.8 Export authorization

Before U. S. companies can sell their bio-engineered products abroad, they must meet U.S. export restrictions. Two independent sets of statutes may apply: the Federal Food, Drug and Cosmetic Act (FD&CA) administered by the Food and Drug Administration (FDA) and the Export Administration Act enforced by the Department of Commerce (DOC).

While FDA review of exports focuses on public health issues, DOC can restrict exports for three entirely different reasons: U. S. foreign policy, short supply of the product in the United States, or national security concerns. For bio-engineered products, the latter justification is most apt to be cited for restricting exports.

Fortunately, most products can be exported freely without obtaining any DOC clearance. Products that are not subject to export restriction are covered by a "general license". This term is a misnomer—there is no such document as a general license. In reality, it means simply that a special DOC license is not required. The export authorization of biotechnology products as administered by FDA will be discussed below.

10.2.8.1 Pre-EC approval

Once FDA has approved a drug or biologic, the FD&CA imposes only minor restrictions on the sale of this product abroad for commercial purposes. The product may lawfully be exported if it meets each of four criteria:

1. The product accords with the specifications of the foreign purchaser;
2. The product does not conflict with the laws of the country to which it is intended for export;
3. The product is labeled on the outside of the shipping package "For Export Only"; and

4. The product is not offered for sale in the United States.

The export situation is different for drugs and biologics that have not yet obtained FDA approval. Unapproved pharmaceutical products can be exported for use in clinical research either at the request of a foreign government or at the request of the manufacturer (as described in 21CFR 312.110).

If the drug or biologic already has an approved investigational new drug (IND) exemption in the United States, the review process is very straightforward. The principal issue then is whether the company has shown that the importing country has approved the shipment. If it has, the export application ordinarily will be approved.

On the other hand, if there is no approved IND, the company must provide information adequate "to satisfy FDA that the drug is appropriate for the proposed investigational use in humans." This information essentially takes the form of a "mini-IND" application. The data in the application are reviewed by the same FDA division that would review a full IND submission for the product. The company also must show that the importing country has approved the export; the FDA will notify that government if the agency approves the request.

The amended Drug Export Amendment Act of 1984 regulations permit foreign governments to submit export requests directly to FDA. These applications do not have to be supported by evidence of safety.

The request to export unapproved pharmaceuticals for clinical trials must include the estimated amount to be used during a specific time, and the export is restricted to that amount. The request should be submitted to the International Affairs Staff at the FDA.

10.2.8.2 Post-EC approval

During the European review process or at least 90 days prior to the date that the applicant proposes to export a drug, an export application request for conditional approval may be submitted (in duplicate) to the Division of Drug Labelling Compliance of the FDA. The Drug Export Amendments Act of 1986 allows export to any of 21 designated countries only if the country has approved the drug. If this condition is met, conditional approval is usually granted. By requesting conditional approval prior to marketing approval in the importing country, export can begin (after submission of approval documents and final labeling) very shortly after final marketing approval.

The export application should contain the following information as specified in the check list below. (This check list is for export of final drug products). References refer to FD&C Act 802.

1. Identify the drug product to be exported [FD&C Act 802(b)(B)(i)].
2. Identify each country to which the drug product is to be exported. These must be included in the list of 21 approved countries specified in [802(b)(4)(A);802(b)(3)(B)(ii)].
3. Name the importer in each country who will receive the drug product. [802(b)(3)(B)(ii)].
4. Include certification by a responsible person of the firm submitting the application that
   (a) the applicant will export the product only to a country listed in [802(b)(4)(A)]. The drug is approved for use in the importing country unless the drug is authorized to be exported under [802(b)(2)]. The applicant will export only those quantities of the drug which may reasonably be sold in each country to which it is to be exported.
   (b) the drug is approved by each country to which it is to be exported unless the drug is authorized to be exported under paragraph (b)(2) and the drug has not been withdrawn from sale in such country [802(b)(3)(B)(iii)(II)]. In addition to the applicant's certification that the drug is approved in the foreign country, a copy of

the approval documents from the foreign country certified by the applicant to be true and accurate is necessary. This certification does not need to be made in the original application but must precede final approval. The documents must be translated to English prior to submission.

(c) the drug is manufactured, processed, packaged, and held in conformity with current good manufacturing practice (cGMP) and is not adulterated under paragraph (a)(I), (a)(2)(A), (a)(3), (c) or (d) of section 501 of the FD&CA. [802(b)(3)(B)(iii)(III)].

(d) the drug will be labeled on the outside of the shipping package with the following statement: "This drug may be sold or offered for sale only in the following countries: _____ ___", the blank spaces being filled with a list of the countries to which export of the drug is authorized under paragraph (4). [802(b)(3)(B)(iii)(IV)] A sample or draft copy of the shipping label intended to be used for the export shipment is requested [802(b)(1)(E)].

(e) an application for approval or licensing of the product in this country has not been disapproved and that the requirements of [801(d)(1)A–D] have been met in that the drug product:
   (1)   accords to the specifications of the foreign purchaser,
   (2)   is not in conflict with the laws of the country to which it is intended for export,
   (3)   is labeled on the outside of the shipping package that it is intended for export and is labeled in accordance with paragraph (1)(E), and
   (4)   is not sold or offered for sale in domestic commerce.

5. Include a certificate by the holder of the exemption or authority for such drug described in paragraph (1)(A) that the holder will actively pursue the approval or licensing of the drug. [802(b)(3)(B)(iv)].

6. Identify the IND exemption number under section 505(i). [802(b)(3)(B)(v)].

7. Identify each establishment in which the drug is manufactured in the United States [802(b)(3)(B)(vi)].

Ten days after FDA receives the application, a notice is published in the *Federal Register* identifying the applicant, product, and countries that are the subjects of the application. If the drug intended for export is manufactured in a facility not yet inspected by FDA, a GMP inspection will take place prior to FDA granting conditional or final approval.

10.2.9 Approval

10.2.9.1 CPMP opinion

As mentioned previously, the CPMP opinion is not binding to the member states. Moreover, the opinion need not be unanimous and can consist of divergent opinions. It is a consensus decision: the opinion can be unanimously negative, unanimously positive, or divergent. The CPMP opinion can be "conditional", tht is, it may be reached with one or more member states stipulating certain conditions, usually involving the provision of further information by the company, before they will effect approval. There is an increasing tendency at the CPMP to include an "approved" Section IB of the dossier (Summary of Product Characteristics) in their final opinion, which should then be used as a guidance for the preparation of the package inserts for the individual countries. The CPMP opinion should be considered as a recommendation to the national authorities.

10.2.9.2 National approvals

The national authorities are required to take the CPMP opinion into due consideration. National authorities can grant conditional marketing authorizations (i.e., require submission of additional information as a prerequisite for granting final approval). Although the member states have to notify the CPMP within 30 days of the issuance of the CPMP opinion of their intended course of action, the subsequent national approval processes may take between one month and one year.

All administrative requirements of the member states must of course be satisfied, including the payment of registration fees and, where applicable, price registration and/or approval. In this stage, the proposed labelling information is also reviewed. These matters must all be resolved strictly with the national authorities.

Since the CPMP opinion has no legal status, it is also possible that member states which have diverged from the CPMP opinion do not follow the CPMP recommendation. In other words, a national authority can still reject the application, despite a positive CPMP opinion. If an applicant wishes to appeal such a rejection, national procedures must be followed.

Once approved, licenses generally must be renewed every five years.

10.2.9.3 Price approvals

In some EC member states, the approval of the dossier is followed by a rather lengthy process—the price regulation process—before marketing authorization is granted. Obtaining price approval is a strictly national procedure, although the prices set in the other member states may be taken into consideration. Current national policies for establishing a price range widely between the member states, reflecting diverse historical approaches to pricing. Four basic control mechanisms are used:

1. Manufacturing costs,
2. Internal market reference,
3. International comparison, and
4. Profit control.

The result is a large difference in prices, ranging from comparatively high prices in West Germany to the lowest prices in Italy and Spain.

It is not the intention of the EC to make individual national systems for drug pricing identical but rather to harmonize the criteria on which pricing decisions can be made. A "Price Transparency" EC directive has been published but has not yet been incorporated in the national legislations.

10.2.10 EC release testing requirements

An applicant can become holder of a marketing authorization only if he has the services of a "qualified person" at his disposal, in accordance with the conditions laid down in the EC directives. This also applies if the applicant imports the drug from a non-EC country into a member state. The directives specify in great detail the minimum conditions of qualification that the qualified person has to fulfill. In practice, the conditions are fulfilled if the qualified person has a university degree in pharmacy and a minimum of two years of practical experience in a pharmaceutical company.

The EC directives specify that the qualified person is responsible for securing:

1. in case of pharmaceuticals manufactured within the EC that each batch of the product has been manufactured and checked in compliance with the laws in force in that member state and in accordance with the requirements of the marketing authorization; or

2. in case of pharmaceuticals coming from non-EC countries that each production batch has undergone in the importing country a full qualitative analysis, quantitative analysis of at least all the active constituents, and all other tests necessary to ensure the quality of the pharmaceutical product in accordance with the requirements of the marketing authorization.

Batches that have undergone such controls in one member state are exempt from the above controls if imported into another member state and accompanied by the control reports signed by the qualified person. The qualified person must certify in writing that each production batch satisfies the above-mentioned provisions.

The EC requirements for release of batches of pharmaceutical products in a member state have been incorporated in the national laws; however, as with other EC provisions, the exact release requirements vary between the countries.

10.2.11   Updates

10.2.11.1   CPMP

Following an opinion of the CPMP, an applicant may wish to apply for a variation in the authorization granted (amendment of the dossier). Applicants are encouraged to submit the same application for variation to all of the member states that have authorized the product, unless there are legitimate reasons for limiting the variation to a limited number of member states.

As for original submissions, the applicant should consult the rapporteur concerning the preparation of the update and the timetable. By definition, the same member state which acted as rapporteur originally should act as rapporteur for the variation.

The update must include a revised Summary of Product Characteristics reflecting the updated information. In addition, the relevant parts of the expert reports must be updated. All members must have received the documentation at least 30 days before the CPMP meeting at which the variation will be discussed.

The rapporteur prepares an assessment report and submits an opinion to the CPMP on whether the proposed variation is major and requires a normal procedure or whether a variation is minor and may undergo an accelerated procedure. If no member state objects, the CPMP adopts at its next meeting the rapporteur's recommendation without discussion. If there is an objection, the CPMP discusses the matter and delivers an opinion as described previously.

If the CPMP delivered a conditional opinion, it can require the applicant to submit an update on certain parts of the dossier at a specified time interval. Again, updates of the relevant pages of the expert reports must be included in the application.

The rapporteur prepares an assessment report of the update and circulates this report to all member states and the CPMP Secretariat. The procedure that follows is essentially identical to the procedure described in section 2.9.

10.2.11.2   National

National authorities can stipulate the condition that the applicant must submit additional information about the product in the future as part of the marketing approval document. Frequently, the update requested by a national authority is also contained in a conditional CPMP opinion. However, a national authority may request additional postregistration information, unrelated to any request made by the CPMP. These matters must be resolved at a strictly national level.

10.3 Issues in the EFTA

As previously mentioned, the EFTA group does not have a unified system for applications for marketing approvals of drugs. The Nordic countries have agreed upon the "Nordic Guidelines". Applications in accordance to the Nordic Guidelines are accepted in Denmark, Iceland, Norway, Finland, and Sweden. Austria and Switzerland have their own rules, but an EC file includes all information necessary and can be submitted both to Austria and Switzerland, after Parts I and V of the file are reformatted.

Within the EFTA countries, certain agreements have been made between countries to accept documentation from each other. There is, for example, the Pharmaceutical Inspection Convention (PIC)—an agreement for mutual recognition of inspections performed of drug manufacturers. Besides the EFTA countries, the following countries honor the PIC agreement: Belgium, Denmark, Germany, United Kingdom, Italy, Liechtenstein, Portugal, Ireland, Romania, and Hungary. An inspection made by the national authorities is honored by the other countries belonging to the PIC Convention, thus eliminating further inspections between the countries.

Another agreement is the Product Evaluation Report (PER) scheme. This agreement provides that drug evaluation reports from one authority can be exchanged with another evaluation authority. Countries belonging to the PER scheme besides the EFTA countries are: Australia, Germany, Hungary, the United Kingdom, Italy, Canada, and the Netherlands.

10.3.1 The Nordic countries

In the development of the Nordic Guidelines issued by the Nordic Council on Medicines (NLN), great care has been taken to meet the guidelines and recommendations of the EC. The structure of the applications for the Nordic countries is identical to the EC structure, but there are differences in detailed registration requirements.

The chemical-pharmaceutical documentation should be introduced with a one to two page synopsis (summary). The synopsis should present the name of the product, the properties of therapeutically active substance, the qualitative and quantitative composition of the finished product, a description of the dosage form and the container, and the name of the manufacturer. This information corresponds to that given in Part IIA of the Notice to Applicants, except that the headings "clinical trial formula" and "development pharmaceutics" are excluded. This specific synopsis should be appended to an EC-formatted dossier for submission in the Nordic countries.

Under the heading "manufacture of the product", the manufacturing chain, the standard of the manufacture, and validation of manufacturing operation should be described in detail. These documents always should be added for the Nordic application if an EC-formatted dossier is used.

The differences in Sections IIC and IID in the guidelines are that the specification and control methods must be signed by a person in charge, and in Sweden it is even a requirement that the original version be submitted. Another difference is that the content of the active substance in the finished product has no specified limit (although usually not more than ±10%), except in Denmark where the EC guidelines are valid (i.e., the limit should be ±5% in the release specification). As far as guidelines for stability studies are concerned, the Nordic Guidelines are generally in agreement with the EC and U. S. FDA guidelines.

There are no requirements for an expert report apart from Denmark. However, the authorities in Norway, Sweden, and Finland appreciate receiving the pharmaceutical export report as an appendix to the chemical-pharmaceutical dossier.

The toxicological and pharmacological documentation closely follow the international scientific guidelines. The same types of studies as in EC and U.S. applications are required, and there must be a rationale for not following the guidelines. The results should be evaluated and presented in a synopsis written so that it may be understood by experts in other disciplines, with references to the original reports. A well-written expert report with proper references to the individual reports can be used as a synopsis. All individual reports must be signed.

The clinical documentation follows the same headings as the Notice to Applicants. The synopsis should be a comprehensive summary describing the human pharmacology and clinical properties of the product. All information given must refer to the individual studies in a reference list. A well-written and referenced expert report can be used as the synopsis. The individual reports should be signed, and a summary of each study should be placed immediately before the study concerned. The format and content of the risk assessment documentation is the same as stated in the Notice to Applicants.

Section V, "Special Particulars", has the same headings as Section V of the Notice to Applicants. One point worth mentioning is that the labeling may be the same in all Nordic countries. Guidelines on how to label proprietary medicinal products in the Nordic countries are available. All Nordic countries have application fees that must be paid for each new preparation, including each new strength of a dosage form.

The manufacturer or an authorized representative applies for the marketing approval of a drug. Applications from foreign manufacturers should be submitted by an authorized representative residing in the country. Denmark does not require an applicant to have a Danish representative if the applicant is based in another EC country. Nordic Guidelines can be obtained from Nordiska Läkemedelsnämnden, Box 607, S-751 25 Uppsala, Sweden.

10.3.2 Austria and Switzerland

Through the PER scheme, Austria and Switzerland exchange such reports with EC countries on already licensed medicines. Approval may be simpler for products already approved in a country belonging to the PER scheme.

In general, the pharmaceutical, preclinical, and clinical information contained in an EC dossier is sufficient for an application in both Austria and Switzerland. However, the Austrian authorities have specific and detailed requirements for the order and format of the general/administrative information and the pharmaceutical data. Use of official forms is obligatory for a large part of the general and administrative data. In addition, the EC expert reports cannot be used; pharmaceutical, preclinical, and clinical expert reports must be prepared in conformity with the Austrian regulations by Austrian experts.

Austrian guidelines, regulations, and forms can be obtained from Österreichischen Staatsdruckerei, (Drucksortenverlag und Verkauf), A-1037 Wien, Rennweg 12a, Austria.

The Swiss drug regulatory authority is called the Interkantonale Kontrollstelle fur Heilmittel (IKS). The IKS accepts EC dossiers; in addition, expert reports in the EC format are accepted, although an adjustment of the layout of the expert reports is required and page-level references must be added.

The standardization of drug regulations in Switzerland has always been something of a problem, mainly because of its federal structure and regulatory differences between the 26 cantons. The working of the Concordat—the treaty of 1900 which established a single approval authority for the whole of Switzerland—has been much improved in recent years, although it still is not fully unified. The IKS Approvals Committee is composed of representatives from university cantons. A supervisory board made up of representatives from 9 of the 26 cantons has a measure of veto over nonscientific aspects of the committee's activities, although there is no cantonal influence on its scientific decisions. Pharmaceutical product approval decisions by the IKS are now, in practice, valid in all the cantons, whereas previously the IKS could only recommend approval to the cantons.

All regulations, guidelines, and forms can be obtained from the IKS at the following address: Interkantonale Kontrollstelle fur Heilmittel, Erlachstrasse 8, CH-3000 Bern 9, Switzerland.

References

[1]   *The Rules Governing Medicinal Products in the European Community: Volume I, The rules governing medicinal products for human use in the European community.* Luxembourg: Office for Official Publications of the European Communities, 1989.

[2]   *The Rules Governing Medicinal Products in the European Community: Volume II, Notice to applicants for marketing authorizations for medicinal products for human use in the Member States of the European Community.* Luxembourg: Office for Official Publications of the European Communities, 1989.

[3]   *The Rules Governing Medicinal Products in the European Community: Volume III, Guidelines on the Quality, Safety and Efficacy of medicinal products for human use (plus Addendum).* Luxembourg: Office for Official Publications of the European Communities, 1989.

[4]   *The Rules Governing Medicinal Products in the European Community: Volume IV, Guide to Good Manufacturing Practice for the manufacture of medicinal products.* Luxembourg: Office for Official Publications of the European Communities, 1989.

[5]   *The Rules Governing Medicinal Products in the European Community: Volume V, The rules governing medicinal products for veterinary use in the European Community.* Luxembourg: Office for Official Publications of the European Communities, 1989. (Volumes I–V can be obtained in the United States from European Community Information Service, 2100 M Street NW, Suite 707, Washington, DC 20037, Tel. (202)862-9500.)

[6]   *Administrative procedures of the Drug Regulatory Authorities in the Nordic Countries.* NLN Publication No. 22.

[7]   *Drug Applications, Nordic Guidelines.* NLN Publications No. 12. (NLN publications can be obtained from Nordiska Läkemedelsnämnden, Box 607, S-751 25 Uppsala, Sweden.)

11 Regulatory issues—Japan

R. H. Rousell and E. L. Greene

Contents

11.1   Introduction

Formalized drug registration schemes have been in place in Japan for approximately 30 years, though the Japanese legislation on pharmaceutical administration dates back to 1889 when regulations on sales of medicines were passed. At first sight, the registration of pharmaceutical products in Japan appears to be extremely complex. However, the process does follow a logical progression. To understand the various issues, it is necessary to know the names and functions of the various organizations involved.

11.2   The Ministry of Health and Welfare

The administrative body responsible for overseeing all aspects of social welfare, social security, and public health is the Ministry of Health and Welfare (MHW) or Koseisho, established on August 10, 1960, as a result of the enactment of the Pharmaceutical Affairs Law (PAL). The MHW consists of home offices and an external body. The home office or Ministry consists of the Minister's Secretariat, nine bureaus, local branches, and affiliated institutions, while the Social Insurance Agency forms the external body.

The Pharmaceutical Affairs Bureau (PAB) is one of the nine bureaus. Other bureaus include the Central Pharmaceutical Affairs Council (CPAC), the Pharmaceutical Affairs Council (PAC), the National Institute of Health (NIH), and the National Institute of Hygienic Sciences (NIHS). The organizational chart for Koseisho is seen in Figure 1 on the next page.

The responsibilities of the Koseisho are contained in nine laws, including the PAL, the law relating to the pharmaceutical industry. The PAL is administered by the Koseisho and regulates all matters relating to the manufacture, import, and sales of pharmaceuticals, cosmetics, and medical devices to ensure their quality, efficacy, and safety, just as the Code of Federal Regulations (CFR) of the Food and Drug Administration (FDA) in the United States. It also covers standards for pharmacy licensing operations and obligations, standards for manufacturer and importer licenses, approval of manufacture and import, as well as reexamination and reevaluation of drugs, licenses for selling drugs and medical devices, and standards and tests for inclusion in the *Japanese Pharmacopeia* (JP) and other official monographs. It includes regulations governing the packaging of drugs, including containers and inserts; regulations on advertising of drugs; requirements for supervision, including inspections; test requirements; orders for improvement as well as cancellation of approvals and licenses; information to be provided in handling of clinical trials; and details of the legal penalties involved with violation of the PAL.

11.2.1   Pharmaceutical Affairs Bureau (PAB)

The PAB supervises both the domestic and foreign based pharmaceutical companies. It is headed by a Director General, a position similar to that of the Commissioner of the FDA in the United States. The PAB is, in turn, composed of eight divisions: Planning, Economic Affairs, First Evaluation and Registration, Second Evaluation and Registration, Pharmaceutical and Chemicals Safety, Inspection and Guidance, Biologics and Antibiotics, and Narcotics. The agency's responsibilities include provision of guidance, encouragement, supervision, and regulations in the following areas:

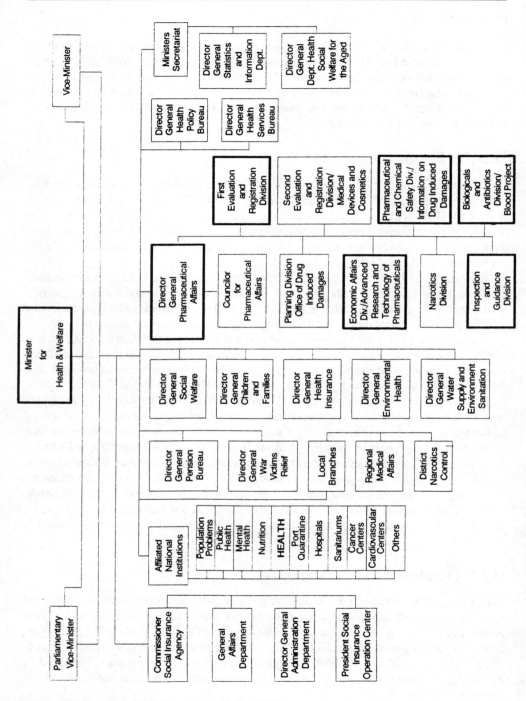

Figure 11.1 Structure of the Ministry of Health and Welfare

1. Testing, examination and research of drugs, quasi-drugs, cosmetics and medical devices;
2. Production, distribution and selling of drugs, quasi-drugs, medical devices and surgical dressings;
3. Overseeing of pharmacists and their activities;
4. Administration of adverse drug reactions suffering relief fund;
5. Control of poisonous and deleterious substances.
6. Enactment and enforcement laws concerning the examination and regulation of chemical substances manufacture;
7. Regulation of adulterated and/or mislabeled products;
8. Regulation of antibiotics and biological product assays;
9. Enforcement of bleeding and blood donor supply service control law;
10. Regulation and control of narcotics and stimulants;
11. Collection of fees on behalf of the Koseisho; and
12. Provision of other services to pharmaceutical manufacturers as may be deemed necessary.

11.2.2 Central Pharmaceutical Affairs Council (CPAC)

The CPAC is probably the most powerful agency within the Ministry. It serves as a government advisory committee whose duties include the recommendation for final approval to manufacture or import all new drugs, as well as to assess periodic drug reevaluation submissions. The agency is responsible for maintaining and revising the JP at least once every ten years. However, given the rapid advances in medicine and pharmaceutical, revisions to the JP are made at approximately five year intervals.

The Committee is composed of approximately 56 regular members and about 400 temporary members. Just as the FDA in the United States may invite various experts to serve on special committees, so the CPAC will draw on their temporary members to serve on various advisory councils, depending upon the degree to which special investigations and deliberations are required. Members of the CPAC serve at the invitation of the Koseisho. Committee assignments are based upon academic specialty and professional field, namely medicine specialties, dentistry, and pharmaceutical or veterinary sciences.

In accordance with Article 4 of the PAL, each prefecture (state in Japan) may establish a local PAC. This local council is under the authority of the governor of the prefecture concerned and acts as a mediator in cooperation with the CPAC in investigating and deliberating pharmaceutical matters essentially of local importance.

11.2.3 NIH and NIHS

The NIH and NIHS have the responsibility for evaluating and approving specifications and test methodology included in drug applications. This includes the practical aspects of the test methodology; the various test methods are set up and performed at the respective institutes.

11.3 Definition of drugs

The PAL Chapter 1, Article 2, defines drugs as follows:

1. Substances/monographs recognized/included in the official JP.
2. Substances intended for use in the diagnosis, cure, or prevention of diseases in humans or animals. These substances do not include equipment or instruments, dental materials, medical supplies, or sanitary materials. They do include substances such as barium sulfate for diagnostic purposes, adrenocortical hormones for therapeutic use, and influenza vaccine for prophylaxis.
3. Substances intended to influence the structure and function of the body of humans or animals. This does not include equipment or instruments used for such purposes.

Drugs are further categorized into ethical and nonprescription drugs. Ethical drugs are intended for use by doctors or dentists and are only available by prescription or under the direction of physicians or dentists. Virtually all such substances are on the National Health Insurance (NHI) price list and can be used under the NHI system. Ethical drugs may not be advertised to the general public. It should be noted that *in vitro* diagnostics are included under the category of pharmaceutical.

Nonprescription drugs are those used for self-medication. They may be purchased directly by the general consumer from a pharmacy or drug store. Usage is at the discretion of the consumer, possibly with advice from the pharmacist.

11.4   Standards for good laboratory practice (GLP), good manufacturing practice (GMP) and good clinical practice (GCP)

Japan has established programs for GLP, GMP, and GCP. These programs are current with the levels of drug quality and clinical testing.

11.4.1   GLP

Essential for the evaluation of a manufacturing/import application for any drug in Japan is the safety test data. To confirm the reliability of such data, the GLP standard for the safety of drugs was established in 1982 and has been in force since April 1983. GLP is also applicable to cases where applications are accompanied by foreign data. Under such circumstances, it is mandatory to attach a GLP certificate issued by the government of the foreign country concerned.

On the basis of bilateral agreements on GLP with several countries, Japan will conduct mutual GLP inspections in order to promote cooperation with the regulatory authorities in such countries and to accelerate mutual acceptance of data conforming to GLP standards.

11.4.2   GMP

In 1987, the MHW issued Notification Number 1051, which dealt with policies on manufacture of drugs by the application of recombinant DNA technology. This directive has stated essentially that the substances produced in this manner for clinical use will be considered new drugs for evaluation by the Committee on Drugs of the CPAC. The regulations were further clarified in Notification Number 11 from the First Division for Evaluation and Registration of the PAB of the Koseisho on 6 June 1988. The directive was issued under the joint signatures of the directors of the First and Second Divisions for Evaluation and Registration and of the Biologics and Anti-biotics Division of the PAB of the MHW.

11.4.3 GCP

The GCP or clinical evaluation guidelines have been prepared for the conduct of clinical trials for individual therapeutic categories. At present there are guidelines on fourteen therapeutic categories. These are:

1. Clinical evaluation of antihypertensives drugs,
2. Evaluation of immunological therapies against malignant tumors,
3. Standardization of indications for antibacterial drugs,
4. Methods for clinical evaluation of analgesics and antiinflammatory drugs,
5. Pediatric drugs,
6. Evaluation of blood preparations, especially plasmapheresis preparations,
7. Evaluation of methods for antiarrhythmic agents,
8. Evaluation of interferon preparations,
9. Clinical evaluation of antiangina pectoris preparations,
10. Clinical evaluation of oral contraceptives,
11. Clinical evaluation of improvers of cerebral circulation and metabolism,
12. Clinical evaluation of antihyperlipemics,
13. Clinical evaluation of anxiolytic drugs, and
14. Evaluation of oral sustained released preparations.

11.5 Registration of drugs

Prior to 1983, any foreign company wishing to market pharmaceutical preparations in Japan needed to form a formal partnership with a Japanese company. The foreign manufacturer could not hold more than 50% partnership in the Japanese company. Thus, up to that time, all pharmaceuticals developed and manufactured by non-Japanese companies were sold in Japan under a license agreement. With the 1983 amendment to the PAL, foreign manufacturers were allowed to apply directly to the Koseisho for approval to import drugs directly into Japan. Previously, while a western manufacturer might have a subsidiary company in Japan, all negotiations with the Koseisho were conducted through the partner Japanese company. Hence, most leading western pharmaceutical manufacturers today do have subsidiary companies in Japan in direct marketing competition with their Japanese counterparts. The laws concerning the functions, structure, and rights of foreign pharmaceutical manufacturers importing drugs into Japan are constantly evolving.

Given a superficial understanding of the Koseisho and the legal processes involved in the activities of the Ministry, the steps involved in seeking approval to manufacture or import a drug substance can be presented. Essentially, there are three steps required prior to marketing. It is first necessary to obtain approval (Shonin) from the Koseisho, then a license (Kyoka) is required for manufacture. Finally, prior to releasing the product onto the market, a price listing must be obtained from the Central Social Medical Insurance Council (Chuikyo).

11.5.1 Registration process

The CPAC consists of 67 committees (Chosakai) and 14 subcommittees. It is headed by an Executive Committee directly supervisory to four main committees: the Committee on Drugs,

Committee on Antibiotics, Committee on Blood Products, and Committee on Biological Products. The Committee on Drugs consists of ten subcommittees: the First Committee on New Drugs, Second Committee on New Drugs, Third Committee on New Drugs, Fourth Committee on New Drugs, Subcommittee on Combination Drugs, Subcommittee on Anticancer Drugs, Subcommittee on Radio-pharmaceutical, Subcommittee on Dental Drugs, Subcommittee on Pesticides, and Subcommittee on Japanese Accepted Names for Drugs. The Committees on Antibiotic Products, on Blood Products, and on Biological Products have only one subcommittee each reporting to them. The organization of the CPAC is seen in Figure 2 opposite.

The entire process involved in the filing and review of the New Drug Application is depicted in Figure 3 on page 180. The applicant sends the NDA to the prefectural governor, who will review it and send it on to the MHW. This may take one to two weeks. The MHW reviews the NDA and sets a date for a one-day hearing (within 6–12 weeks of the receipt of the dossier). One week before the hearing, the PAB will notify the applicant of what will be discussed at the hearing. On the morning of the hearing, the file will be checked for completeness; in the afternoon, there is a check of the raw data, usually two clinical parts and one pharmacology part. At the hearing, the applicant will receive instructions or questions, or both, to which responses are required. The time to clear this stage of the process is dependent on how quickly the company responds to the requests and for the information to be exchanged.

If the drug is a new one, then special deliberations are held to address the innovative aspects. The NIHS checks the test methods in the application as well as the active substance itself; this may take three months. Concurrently, the MHW holds a GLP inspection and sends the results to the GLP Evaluation Committee. The applicant is notified of the results of the inspection.

About two months after all of the instructions have been addressed and the questions answered, the file is registered and given to the CPAC Committee on New Drugs (Chosakai) for review. The experts may give instructions on designated items to the applicant, whose compliance is mandatory. A loop may be formed, and the time needed will be a function of how long it takes for resolution of the concerns of the Chosakai. Generally, it is three to six months.

After being checked for completeness, the dossier is registered and again sent to the Chosakai for review. The Subcommittee reports to the appropriate Committee on Drugs, which then reviews and reports back to the Executive Committee. The Executive Committee then makes its recommendation to the Minister of Health.

The applicant learns from the prefectural governor of the approval; the applicant deals directly with the prefecture. The product may be sold, but it will not be prescribed since reimbursement cannot take place until a price is assigned by the NHI.

The total time involved, aside from that required to respond to instructions and questions, is a function of the dates of the various committees' meetings. They are usually quarterly, so if an applicant just misses a session, three months may be lost until the committee sits again.

11.5.2 Data required

The data required to submit an application for approval of drugs produced by cell culture are defined by the 1987/1988 directives from the Koseisho. A useful rule of thumb is that the requirements are based to a great extent on precedent. This means that if a similar product has been studied previously and an application for approval and license of drugs (NDA) filed and subsequently approved, then the same procedures and data will have to be collected for the new product. An exception is naturally made if it can be shown that an experiment undertaken for the

CENTRAL PHARMACEUTICAL AFFAIRS COUNCIL

COMMITTEES AND SUBCOMMITTEES

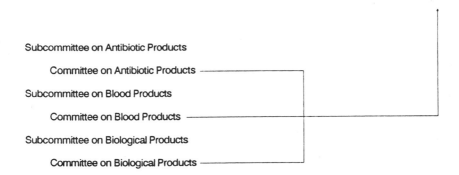

First Subcommittee on new Drugs

Second Subcommittee on New Drugs

Third Subcommittee on New Drugs

Subcommittee on Combination Drugs

Subcommittee on Anticancer Drugs   Committee on Drugs

Subcommittee on Radiopharmaceuticals

Subcommitte on Dental Drugs

Subcommittee on Pesticides

Subcommittte on Japanese Accepted Names for Drugs

EXECUTIVE COMMITTEE

Subcommittee on Antibiotic Products

Committee on Antibiotic Products

Subcommittee on Blood Products

Committee on Blood Products

Subcommittee on Biological Products

Committee on Biological Products

Figure 11.2   CPAC committees (Chosakai) and subcommittees

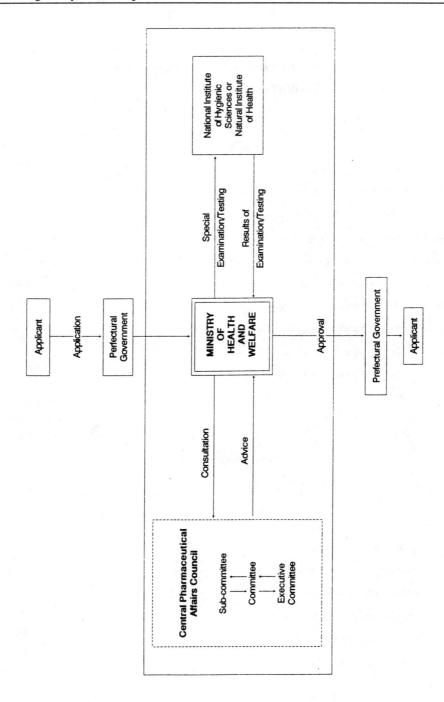

Figure 11.3 Licensing review process

previous/competitor product was completely irrelevant. An explanation then can be offered as to the valid reasons why the particular procedure was not repeated for the new preparation.

At relatively frequent intervals, the PAB publishes details of all regulatory requirements for licensing drugs in Japan. The 1988 volume, "Drug Registration Requirements in Japan", is known as the Red Book because of the color of its cover. The third edition was issued in August 1988, at which time guidelines for drugs whose active ingredients are peptides or proteins produced by cell culture were being formulated in Japan. A fourth edition, the Blue Book, was released in late 1991. It contains the specific information on peptides or proteins produced by new technologies such as genetically engineered preparations or monoclonal antibodies. Many of the more general requirements remain unchanged. This review of the various requirements is based upon Notification Number 11 issued by the First Division for Evaluation and Registration of the PAB of the Koseisho in June 6, 1988, under the joint signatures of the directors of the First and Second Divisions for Evaluation and Registration and of the Biologics and Antibiotics Division of the PAB of the Koseisho.

11.5.2.1 Definition of terms

CELL CULTURE TECHNIQUE: The technique for manufacturing gene products by cultivating human or animal cells containing structural genes encoding the target molecules.

SEED CELL LINES: Cell lines established and used as materials for producing drugs.

MASTER CELL BANKS (MCB):   Cells obtained by proliferation of the seed lines for the duration of the fewest passages under specified conditions and then filling the master cells banks into appropriate ampules.

CELL BANKS: Cells for production obtained by pooling one or more ampules of the MCBs, and further cultivation of the resultant cell suspensions under specified conditions ultimately filling them into appropriate ampules.

It should be noted that because of the recent and innovative nature of production of drugs through these new biotechnology procedures, the CPAC considered that such preparations should be regulated as entirely new drugs. This means that even though an existing product prepared by purification of animal/human tissues or fluids (e.g., porcine derived insulin or plasma derived factor VIII) is already available in Japan, the genetically engineered products must undergo complete preclinical and clinical testing through all phases of their development.

11.5.2.2 Manufacturing information

As with the conventional biological preparations, information on in-process quality assurance (QA) of manufacturing procedures is required at appropriate stages.

1. The origin and characteristics of the seed cell line must be defined, giving as much information as possible on the origin, establishment and passage history.
2. Characteristics of the seed cell lines covering morphology, growth cytogenetics, immunological phenotype, isozyme, presence of viral genome, oncogenicity and productivity of the target product must be described in full detail.
3. The methods of preparation, storage, and maintenance of the MCB should be defined. QA relating to the stability of the MCB is an obvious necessity.
4. Methods of preparation, storage, and maintenance of the cell bank for production and the QA of such must be dealt with.
5. With cells grown beyond the ordinary condition for manufacturing drugs, the stability of the cells must be examined.

6. The cell culture condition at each stage must be defined.
7. The absence of contaminants, such as bacteria, mycoplasma, and fungi, must be confirmed for all the stages. For cells at stages 1. and 2. above, the absence of viruses possible in the animal species from which the cells are derived must be confirmed. Reasons for exceptions to such procedures must be supplied in detail. If animals are used to grow the cells, the absence of viruses which might be expected in the animals should be confirmed in the cells at stage 3. As a general principal, cells with potential of harboring viruses likely to be pathogenic to human should not be used.
8. The presence or absence of such endogenous pathogens such as retroviruses should be confirmed for cells at stages 1. and 2. using methodology such as reverse transcriptase activity assays and electron microscopy. Furthermore, such assays should also be performed on cells which have undergone standard induction treatments.
9. The procedures for the isolation and purification of the desired target product must be covered. For this purpose a production flow chart is preferred. The procedure and efficiency of separating the target product from impurities such as contaminating proteins and DNA should be specified. If freedom from viral contamination of the target product as a result of the use of viruses during production or the presence of endogenous virus in the seed cell line or other parts of the manufacture cannot be confirmed, the procedure and efficacy of inactivation/removal of such viruses must be specified. Finally, the absence of retroviruses by means of hybridization methods should be proven in the target products. For human antibodies, the absence of Epstein-Barr viral DNA must be demonstrated. If animals are used to grow the cells in production, the absence of viruses which may be derived from such animals and find their way into the target product must be confirmed.

11.5.2.3   Structure determination, physicochemical, and other final product properties

QA testing plays a major role in this area, not only during the developmental phases but also to confirm that the product remains the same from batch to batch. The essential features are:

1. Structural Properties: The chemical structure and composition of the active ingredient should be defined in as much detail as possible. Not all the items may be suitable or indeed necessary for repeated QA release testing but, of course, may be warranted at specified intervals on random lots to confirm that the production method has remained stable. The items of importance are:
   a.   amino acid composition,
   b.   amino acid sequence,
   c.   terminal amino acids,
   d.   positioning of any disulfide bonds, and
   e.   dipeptide analysis.
   For substances of very high molecular weight, the terminal amino acid sequences should be determined as far as possible.
2. Physicochemical Properties   The following may be important:
   a.   spectrophotometric properties (i.e., UV absorption),
   b.   electrophoretic mobility (i.e., polyacrylamide gel electrophoresis),
   c.   isoelectric point utilizing (i.e., gel isoelectric focusing),
   d.   molecular weight (i.e., SDS gel electrophoresis),

  e. liquid chromatography, or

  f. superstructure (i.e., circular dichroism).

3. Immunochemical Properties The immunochemical properties of the active ingredient which are used for identification, purity determination, and quantitative assays must be detailed. For example, the reaction between the active ingredient and specific antibodies directed against it should be confirmed using standard methods such as immunoassays or immunoelectrophoresis.

4. Biological Properties: The properties of importance relating specifically to the activity of the product concerned must be defined. Items to be covered include:

  a. biological activities and purity (i.e., specific activity);

  b. in the case of enzymes, their enzymatic activity;

  c. for monoclonal antibodies, properties inherent in the antigen-antibody reaction should be targeted, including interaction with specific antigen, cross-reactivity with pseudoantigens and histological affinity; and

  d. in the event of multiple target cells in the biological effects of the active ingredients, specific activities should be chosen and clearly defined.

5. Sugar composition

6. For immunoglobulins, the class and subclass should be characterized.

11.5.2.4 QA specifications and assay methods

Detailed specifications and assay methods must be established so that the characteristics of the cell culture drug may be accurately reflected. The following items should be covered:

1. Origin: It must be clearly stated that the product is a cell culture drug.

2. The appearance, solubility, crystallinity, and stability, including hygroscopic activity, must be covered.

3. Identification: Appropriate methods, including physicochemical tests, bioassays, and immunoassays, should be applied.

4. Constituent amino acids.

5. A peptide map may be required.

6. Sugar Content

7. Purity Testing: The same tests which might be required for ordinary drugs should be performed. In addition, with drugs where tolerance limits have been established for DNA, polypeptides, other proteins, degradation products, or other substances which may be derived from the cells, the culture medium or the production methodology, it is necessary to perform appropriate testing using liquid chromatography, immunoassays, DNA hybridization, or other relevant tests.

8. Similar testing should be performed for such substances which might be derived from the cell culture media using liquid chromatography, immunoassays, DNA hybridization or other appropriate methods. Testing for heavy metals or arsenic should be established if appropriate, considering the production methodology and intended dosage and route of administration.

9. Loss on drying and moisture determination. Limits should be established, defined and maintained.

10. Residue on ignition: If appropriate, this should be defined and established.

11. Biological activity: As physicochemical testing in isolation may not serve, in many instances, to ensure the identification, purity and titer of the complex substances derived

from body tissues and fluids and now manufactured by culture techniques, it may be necessary to utilize bioassays for specialized performance characterizations. For monoclonal antibodies, for example, appropriate antigen specificity tests and complement fixation, where appropriate, should be evaluated.

12. Pyrogen testing.
13. Quantitative assays. Either physicochemical or bioassays should be established for quantitation. If physicochemical methods are adopted, it is necessary to confirm linearity between the physicochemical assay and the bioassay.

11.5.2.5 Clinical information

Prior to commencing clinical trials on any new drug, it is necessary to submit a clinical trial plan to the MHW. The clinical trial plan should be accompanied by sufficient information on product characteristics, stability, toxicity, and preclinical testing to indicate that studies in humans are appropriate and may be conducted with a satisfactory therapeutic margin and safety in relation to the disease condition under investigation. However, to submit an NDA, a great deal more preclinical, manufacturing, QA, and stability data must accompany the results of the clinical studies. Animal research, quality assurance and stability data may proceed in parallel with the clinical studies. Indeed, even changes in manufacturing processes are possible at this stage, provided there is no alteration to the therapeutically or physiologically active components in the study drug formulation. On this basis, it is essential that when the NDA is filed, all such data are complete and included in the application. In addition, foreign companies must designate an in-country caretaker (who may be a member of the subsidiary company) to act on their behalf and take preventive measures against possible harmful effects on human health and hygiene, in as much as foreign manufacturers do not have the means to do so.

11.5.3 Stability

During drug development and clinical testing, stability studies are essential. Japanese regulations are very specific in this context. They define:

1. the number of lots of each vial size to be studied (It is usual to require three different lots of each vial size.);
2. the exact tests to be performed;
3. the exact frequency of such testing;
4. the number of different vials to be studied at each test at each time point and the repeats required for each sample (usually in triplicate); and
5. the storage conditions under which the vials must be maintained during throughout the duration of the stability experiment.

The storage condition is defined in accordance with the eventual recommended storage conditions for the licensed/marketed product. The regulations require worst case storage conditions in each instance, usually ±1 °C of the worst case temperature. Accelerated stability studies may be approved in certain instances under specific conditions. Here, too, the requirements of such accelerated storage conditions are carefully defined.

For any particular application for a shelf life of a particular drug, the Japanese regulations require satisfactory stability testing to be proven for at least six months beyond the requested shelf life.

11.5.4   Toxicological Studies

Such studies do not constitute QA release requirements. However, they are essential for filing of the NDA in Japan. The nature and extent of such toxicological studies may only be decided on an individual case basis considering the diversity of characteristics and clinical administration of drugs manufactured through the new bioculture techniques. It is necessary to give the rationale for selecting any particular toxicological model. As further knowledge in this field is gained, so further regulations may come into force. The guidelines presented in the sections below apply.

11.5.4.1   General precautions

The toxicological studies must be rationally performed considering the method of production, physicochemical properties, pharmacological activity, mechanism of action, pharmacokinetics, indications, dosage, and administration of the drug in question. The nature and content of impurities, their relation to the active ingredients, and the effects of excipient should be taken into account and covered when interpreting the results. Naturally, as with any product, the ideal situation is to remove the impurities during the course of production.

The animal species chosen should be such that positive controls may be defined. In other words, if a drug is expected to demonstrate any form of toxicity, the animal species chosen must be susceptible to such toxic manifestations. In surrogate toxicity and reproduction studies, this is especially important. Accordingly, the reason for choosing any particular test species should be stated.

The route, frequency, and duration of administration must be based on the intended clinical administration. With repeated doses in animal toxicological studies, antibody production should be evaluated after such administration. The influence of antibody production on the pharmacological effects must be considered. The specificity of the antibody to a particular antigen/epitope must be evaluated. Obviously, wherever possible, it is preferable to choose an animal species in which antigenicity is likely to be no more of a problem than it might be in man.

Parts of the toxicological studies may be omitted provided the active ingredient of the cell culture drug can be demonstrated to be identical to the human-derived substance studied in previous toxicological experiments. However, it is necessary to evaluate the toxicity of impurities in detail. Wherever possible, existing guidelines for toxicity studies should be followed.

11.5.4.2   Types of toxicological studies

1. Acute Toxicity: These are essential and should be performed in at least two animal species, including one rodent.
2. Subacute Toxicity: Such studies are also required, except in instances such as vaccines where the frequency and duration of intended clinical administration in man are limited. It may be necessary to limit the duration of the study because of antibody production. The reasons for such limitations should be given.
3. Chronic Toxicity: If possible, such studies should be performed. Again, antibody production may preclude chronic toxicity studies, in which event the reasons for omission must be stated.
4. Reproductive Studies: If such studies are omitted, the reasons must be stated.
5. Mutagenicity Studies: If appropriate, such testing should be conducted using mammalian cultured cells initially. If findings suggest mutagenicity, further *in vivo* studies must be carried out.

6. Carcinogenicity studies: If such studies are omitted the reasons for such omission must be stated.
7. Dependency and local irritation: Relevant studies should be conducted.
8. Antigenicity studies: Such studies are essential where the culture drug concerned will be administered for long periods of time or when it contains ingredients different from the human-derived counterpart, which may elicit antibody responses. Where there are valid reasons, such studies may be omitted.
9. Pyrogen: While pyrogen testing is conventionally performed in rabbits, additional methods for detecting pyrogenicity are encouraged.
10. Miscellaneous: The biological activities of the culture drug must be considered in relation to any particular toxicity tests or animal models selected. For example, when evaluating AIDS drugs whose toxicity is expected to relate to immune function, testing should be focused on immunological toxicity.

11.5.5 Pharmacological studies

These studies should be carried out in animals in the same manner as for conventional new drugs.

11.5.5.1 Basic pharmacology

If the active ingredient of the cell culture drug is confirmed to be identical to that of the body-derived substance that has already been studied pharmacologically, such studies may be omitted except for:

1. Basic pharmacological studies on efficacy, including comparative studies with the analogous drug of body origin.
2. Confirmatory studies to verify identity in superstructure with a body-derived analogous drug such as binding, bound state, and affinity for receptors; biological effects on multiple target cells, if any, for vaccines, immunogenicity, and interactions with antibodies.

11.5.5.2 Absorption, distribution, metabolism and excretion

These studies should be carried out in appropriate animal models. Comparison with the conventional body-derived drugs may be useful, if available.

1. Absorption: The following recommendations are supplied for guidance:
   a.   quantitative assays should be performed ideally utilizing two different methods, one of which should be a bioassay;
   b.   the results of administration must be the same as that intended in clinical use for the marketed drug; and
   c.   single and repeated dose studies are essential. The pattern of blood levels should be clarified at several dose levels and parameters such as half-life, area under the curve (AUC), C_{Max} and T_{Max} should be calculated.
2. Distribution: In principle, this should be evaluated by examination of the main organs, after both single and repeated doses. Potential accumulation should be discussed based upon data obtained after repeated doses. If the target organ is known, it is advisable to examine the distribution within such organs.
3. Metabolism: The metabolism and levels of metabolites in the blood and urine should be determined. If this is impossible, *in vitro* data from which the rates and sites of

metabolism may be assumed are necessary. These requirements are especially important for drugs that manifest their effects after being metabolized and where the metabolites themselves possess biological activity.

4. Excretion: Information on excretion should be obtained by evaluation of equivalence between cell culture-derived drug and the conventional body-derived preparation.

If there already is an approved cell culture drug with the same active ingredients, formulation, dosage, and administration for which a substantial amount of data on absorption, distribution, metabolism, and excretion is available, it is only required to submit data confirming the equivalence between the new cell culture drug and the approved one. In such instances, it is necessary to prove the equivalence using the proper animals prior to proceeding to human studies.

11.6   Clinical studies

Conventional Phase I, II, and III studies must be carefully performed and the results evaluated after completion of each phase before proceeding to the next phase.

11.6.1   Phase I studies

During Phase I, conventional pharmacological studies should be conducted covering pharmacokinetics and pharmacodynamics. The pharmacokinetics involve the usual evaluation of absorption, distribution, metabolism, and excretion. Pharmacodynamics cover the physiologic and/or toxicologic changes which may be induced by the drug in any body system. Single and repeat dose studies are required. While Phase I studies with conventional drugs are often conducted in normal, nonpatient volunteers, this is usually not the case with biological drugs derived either from cell culture or from animal/human tissues/organs/body fluids. Phase I studies usually utilize actual patients who are in a relatively quiescent/stable state as regards their disease processes.

11.6.2   Phase II studies

Phase II studies are indeed intensive studies of therapeutic activity and safety in small groups of patients before proceeding to large-scale Phase III studies of efficacy and safety.

11.6.3   Phase III studies

In clinical studies, special attention should be paid to:
1. local and systemic allergic reactions;
2. antibody production, defining and characterizing antibodies produced against ingredients in the cell culture drug and to induction of autoantibodies directed against host antigens;
3. local reactions at application sites;
4. alterations in pharmacokinetics and any possible alterations in drug activity as a result of interactions with antibodies; and
5. pyrogenicity.

In all instances, where practical, comparisons against conventional body-derived drugs already on the market should be made. Changes in antibodies and in drug effects should be observed and compared; similarly, comparative studies of the expected treatment periods are desirable utilizing the appropriate types (age, height, weight, sex, and other demographic parameters) and numbers of patients.

11.7 Conclusion

This overview has attempted to define the necessary steps to register a new technology product in Japan, emphasizing wherever possible the role of QA. Comprehensive guidelines are published by the Koseisho in the fourth (most recent) edition of "Drug Registration Requirements in Japan". The English version was released in October 1991 and, in accordance with the blue cover, is known as the Blue Book. The requirements for the registration process rely to a tremendous degree on precedent and on the studies performed in the past with similar drugs. Biotechnology products such as the genetically engineered or the monoclonal preparations produced by cell culture are considered as entirely new products and must undergo complete and comprehensive studies, many of which, of course, may be based upon past experience with similar products manufactured from human/animal body tissues/organs/fluids.

Careful attention must always be paid to the limits for any specification or parameter studied. Thus, the allowable limits for a concentration is ±10% of the mean; where temperature ranges are defined, the worst case should be utilized, again with only a deviation from the worst case of ±1 °C; for room temperature storage, the actual definition of room temperature must be used.

These few examples attempt to emphasize the importance of following the defined requirements to the letter. There is very little room for negotiation and, even then, an excellent reason with complete data must be available to allow any chance of waiving or modifying the particular requirement. Finally, the importance of following precedent cannot be overstressed; if a similar drug was studied and licensed previously, the same testing procedures throughout should be followed.

Japan is one of the active participants in the movement towards harmonization of regulatory requirements (as represented by the International Conference on Harmonization) and, as such, has already taken steps to this end. There are plans for the publication, in Japanese and English, of a Summary Basis of Approval. Analysis of GCP began in April 1992; toxicity testing requirements, etc. are being changed. Further positive results are expected as a result of this endeavor.

References

[1] *Drug Registration Requirement in Japan*, 4th Edition. Yakuji Nippo, Ltd., 1991.
[2] Greene, E. "The Regulatory Process in Japan." *Regulatory Affairs 2* (1990): 243–260.

Abbreviations

ACS	American Chemical Society
BCA	bicinchoninic acid
BI	biological indicators
BLI-LS	Biosafety Level 1 large-scale
CAS	chemical abstract number
CBER	Center for Biologics Evaluation and Research
CEO	Chief executive officer
CERCL	Comprehensive Environmental Response, Compensation, and Liability Act
CFR	Code of Federal Regulations
cGMP	current good manufacturing practice
C_p	capability index
CPAC	Central Pharmaceutical Affairs Council
C_{pk}	process capability index
CSO	Consumer safety officer
CV	coefficient of variance
DEHP	diethylhexylphthalate
DMF	Drug master file
DOC	Department of Commerce
DOT	Department of Transportation
DW	distilled water
EC	European Economic Community
EFTA	European Free Trade Association
EHS	environmental health and safety
ELA	Establishment License Application
ELISA	enzyme-linked immunosorbent assay
EPA	Environmental Protection Agency
EPCRA	Emergency Planning and Community Right-to-know Amendment
ERT	emergency response team
ESA	emission spectrographic analysis
EtO	ethylene oxide
EU	endotoxin units
FDA	Food and Drug Administration
FD&CA	Food, Drug, and Cosmetic Act
FMOC	9-fluorenylmethyl-chloro formate
GC	gas chromatography
GLP	good laboratory practice
GMP	good manufacturing practice
HPLC	high-performance liquid chromatography
IDE	Investigational Device Exemption (application)

IKS	Interkantonale Kontrolstelle für Heilmittel
IND	Investigational New Drug (application)
IPP	Injury Prevention Plan
IQ	installation quality
IR	infrared
IRB	Institutional Review Board
IRMA	immunoradiometric assay
JP	Japanese Pharmacopeia
LAL	limulus amebocyte lysate
MCB	master cell bank
MHW	Ministry of Health and Welfare
MWCB	manufacturer's working cell bank
NBD	4-chloro-7-nitrobenzofuran
NDA	New Drug Application
NF	National Formulary
NHI	National Health Insurance
NIH	National Institutes of Health
NIHS	National Institute of Hygienic Sciences
NLN	Nordic Council on Medicines
NRC	Nuclear Regulatory Commission
OJT	on-the-job training
OPA	o-phthalidialdehyde
OQ	operational quality
OSHA	Occupational Safety and Health Administration
PAB	Pharmaceutical Affairs Bureau
PAC	Pharmaceutical Affairs Council
PAL	Pharmaceutical Affairs Law
PDA	Parenteral Drug Association
PDL	population doubling level
PER	Product Evaluation Report
pg	picograms
PHS	Public Health Service
Ph Eur	European Pharmacopeia
pI	isoelectric point
PIC	Pharmaceutical Inspection Convention
PLA	Product License Application
PLC	programmable logic controllers
PMA	Pre-Market Approval (application)
ppm	parts per million
PQ	performance quality
PTH	phenylthiohydantin
PVC	polyvinylchloride

QA	quality assurance
QC	quality control
R&D	research and development
RCRA	Resource Conservation and Recovery Act
RIA	radioimmunoassay
ROI	residue on ignition
SARA	Superfund Amendments and Reauthorization
SDS-PAGE	sodium dodecyl sulfate-polyacrylamide gel electrophoresis
SIP	steam-in-place
SLR	spore log reduction
SOP	standard operating procedure
SPC	statistical process control
SS	sum of squares
TCF	tissue culture fluid
TLC	thin-layer chromatography
TSDF	treatment, storage, and disposal facility
USP	United States Pharmacopeia
WFI	water for injection

Appendices

Appendix I: For Z values—Areas of a standard normal distribution

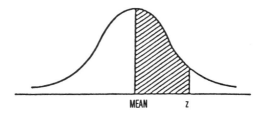

MEAN   Z

Table of areas from mean to distances Z

Z	.00	.01	.02	.03	.04	.05	.06	.07	.08	.09
0.0 0000	.0040	.0080	.0120	.0160	.0199	.0239	.0279	.0319	.0359
0.1 0398	.0438	.0478	.0517	.0557	.0596	.0636	.0675	.0714	.0753
0.2 0793	.0832	.0871	.0910	.0948	.0987	.1026	.1064	.1103	.1141
0.3 1179	.1217	.1255	.1293	.1331	.1368	.1406	.1443	.1480	.1517
0.4 1554	.1591	.1628	.1664	.1700	.1736	.1772	.1808	.1844	.1879
0.5 1915	.1950	.1985	.2019	.2054	.2088	.2123	.2157	.2190	.2224
0.6 2257	.2291	.2324	.2357	.2389	.2422	.2454	.2486	.2518	.2549
0.7 2580	.2612	.2642	.2673	.2704	.2734	.2764	.2794	.2823	.2852
0.8 2881	.2910	.2939	.2967	.2995	.3023	.3051	.3078	.3106	.3133
0.9 3159	.3186	.3212	.3238	.3264	.3289	.3315	.3340	.3365	.3389
1.0 3413	.3438	.3461	.3485	.3508	.3531	.3554	.3577	.3599	.3621
1.1 3643	.3665	.3686	.3708	.3729	.3749	.3770	.3790	.3810	.3830
1.2 3849	.3869	.3888	.3907	.3925	.3944	.3962	.3980	.3997	.4015
1.3 4032	.4049	.4066	.4082	.4099	.4115	.4131	.4147	.4162	.4177
1.4 4192	.4207	.4222	.4236	.4251	.4265	.4279	.4292	.4306	.4319
1.5 4332	.4345	.4357	.4370	.4382	.4394	.4406	.4418	.4429	.4441
1.6 4452	.4463	.4474	.4484	.4495	.4505	.4515	.4525	.4535	.4545
1.7 4554	.4564	.4573	.4582	.4591	.4599	.4608	.4616	.4625	.4633
1.8 4641	.4649	.4656	.4664	.4671	.4678	.4686	.4693	.4699	.4706
1.9 4713	.4719	.4726	.4732	.4738	.4744	.4750	.4756	.4761	.4767
2.0 4772	.4778	.4783	.4788	.4793	.4898	.4803	.4808	.4812	.4817
2.1 4821	.4826	.4830	.4834	.4838	.4842	.4846	.4850	.4854	.4857
2.2 4861	.4864	.4868	.4871	.4875	.4878	.4881	.4884	.4887	.4890
2.3 4893	.4896	.4898	.4901	.4904	.4906	.4909	.4911	.4913	.4916
2.4 4918	.4920	.4922	.4925	.4927	.4929	.4931	.4932	.4934	.4936
2.5 4938	.4940	.4941	.4943	.4945	.4946	.4948	.4949	.4951	.4952
2.6 4953	.4955	.4956	.4957	.4959	.4960	.4961	.4962	.4963	.4964
2.7 4965	.4966	.4967	.4968	.4969	.4970	.4971	.4972	.4973	.4974
2.8 4974	.4975	.4976	.4977	.4977	.4978	.4979	.4979	.4980	.4981
2.9 4981	.4982	.4982	.4983	.4984	.4984	.4985	.4985	.4986	.4986
3.0 49865	.4987	.4987	.4988	.4988	.4989	.4989	.4989	.4990	.4990
4.0 4999683									

Appendix II: F-distribution ($\alpha = .05$)

F_2 \ F_1	1	2	3	4	5	6	7	8	9	10	12	15	20	24	30	40	60	120	∞
1	161.45	199.50	215.71	224.58	230.16	233.99	236.77	238.88	240.54	241.88	243.91	245.95	248.01	249.05	250.09	251.14	252.20	253.25	254.32
2	18.513	19.000	19.164	19.247	19.296	19.330	19.353	19.371	19.385	19.396	19.413	19.429	19.446	19.454	19.462	19.471	19.479	19.487	19.496
3	10.128	9.5521	9.2766	9.1172	9.0135	8.9406	8.8868	8.8452	8.8123	8.7855	8.7446	8.7029	8.6602	8.6385	8.6166	8.5944	8.5720	8.5494	8.5265
4	7.7086	6.9443	6.5914	6.3883	6.2560	6.1631	6.0942	6.0410	5.9988	5.9644	5.9117	5.8578	5.8025	5.7744	5.7459	5.7170	5.6878	5.6581	5.6281
5	6.6079	5.7861	5.4095	5.1922	5.0503	4.9503	4.8759	4.8183	4.7725	4.7351	4.6777	4.6188	4.5581	4.5272	4.4957	4.4638	4.4314	4.3984	4.3650
6	5.9874	5.1433	4.7571	4.5337	4.3874	4.2839	4.2066	4.1468	4.0990	4.0600	3.9999	3.9381	3.8742	3.8415	3.8082	3.7743	3.7398	3.7047	3.6688
7	5.5914	4.7374	4.3468	4.1203	3.9715	3.8660	3.7870	3.7257	3.6767	3.6365	3.5747	3.5108	3.4445	3.4105	3.3758	3.3404	3.3043	3.2674	3.2298
8	5.3177	4.4590	4.0662	3.8378	3.6875	3.5806	3.5005	3.4381	3.3881	3.3472	3.2840	3.2184	3.1503	3.1152	3.0794	3.0428	3.0053	2.9669	2.9276
9	5.1174	4.2565	3.8626	3.6331	3.4817	3.3738	3.2927	3.2296	3.1789	3.1373	3.0729	3.0061	2.9365	2.9005	2.8637	2.8259	2.7872	2.7475	2.7067
10	4.9646	4.1028	3.7083	3.4780	3.3258	3.2172	3.1355	3.0717	3.0204	2.9782	2.9130	2.8450	2.7740	2.7372	2.6996	2.6609	2.6211	2.5801	2.5379
11	4.8443	3.9823	3.5874	3.3567	3.2039	3.0946	3.0123	2.9480	2.8962	2.8536	2.7876	2.7186	2.6464	2.6090	2.5705	2.5309	2.4901	2.4480	2.4045
12	4.7472	3.8853	3.4903	3.2592	3.1059	2.9961	2.9134	2.8486	2.7964	2.7534	2.6866	2.6169	2.5436	2.5055	2.4663	2.4259	2.3842	2.3410	2.2962
13	4.6672	3.8056	3.4105	3.1791	3.0254	2.9153	2.8321	2.7669	2.7144	2.6710	2.6037	2.5331	2.4589	2.4202	2.3803	2.3392	2.2966	2.2524	2.2064
14	4.6001	3.7389	3.3439	3.1122	2.9582	2.8477	2.7642	2.6987	2.6458	2.6021	2.5342	2.4630	2.3879	2.3487	2.3082	2.2664	2.2230	2.1778	2.1307
15	4.5431	3.6823	3.2874	3.0556	2.9013	2.7905	2.7066	2.6408	2.5876	2.5437	2.4753	2.4035	2.3275	2.2878	2.2468	2.2043	2.1601	2.1141	2.0658
16	4.4940	3.6337	3.2389	3.0069	2.8524	2.7413	2.6572	2.5911	2.5377	2.4935	2.4247	2.3522	2.2756	2.2354	2.1938	2.1507	2.1058	2.0589	2.0096
17	4.4513	3.5915	3.1968	2.9647	2.8100	2.6987	2.6143	2.5480	2.4943	2.4499	2.3807	2.3077	2.2304	2.1898	2.1477	2.1040	2.0584	2.0107	1.9604
18	4.4139	3.5546	3.1599	2.9277	2.7729	2.6613	2.5767	2.5102	2.4563	2.4117	2.3421	2.2686	2.1906	2.1497	2.1071	2.0629	2.0166	1.9681	1.9168
19	4.3808	3.5219	3.1274	2.8951	2.7401	2.6283	2.5435	2.4768	2.4227	2.3779	2.3080	2.2341	2.1555	2.1141	2.0712	2.0264	1.9796	1.9302	1.8780
20	4.3513	3.4928	3.0984	2.8661	2.7109	2.5990	2.5140	2.4471	2.3928	2.3479	2.2776	2.2033	2.1242	2.0825	2.0391	1.9938	1.9464	1.8963	1.8432
21	4.3248	3.4668	3.0725	2.8401	2.6848	2.5757	2.4876	2.4205	2.3661	2.3210	2.2504	2.1757	2.0960	2.0540	2.0102	1.9645	1.9165	1.8657	1.8117
22	4.3009	3.4434	3.0491	2.8167	2.6613	2.5491	2.4638	2.3965	2.3419	2.2967	2.2258	2.1508	2.0707	2.0283	1.9842	1.9380	1.8895	1.8380	1.7831
23	4.2793	3.4221	3.0280	2.7955	2.6400	2.5277	2.4422	2.3748	2.3201	2.2747	2.2036	2.1282	2.0476	2.0050	1.9605	1.9139	1.8649	1.8128	1.7570
24	4.2597	3.4028	3.0088	2.7763	2.6207	2.5082	2.4226	2.3551	2.3002	2.2547	2.1834	2.1077	2.0267	1.9838	1.9390	1.8920	1.8424	1.7897	1.7331
25	4.2417	3.3852	2.9912	2.7587	2.6030	2.4904	2.4047	2.3371	2.2821	2.2365	2.1649	2.0889	2.0075	1.9643	1.9192	1.8718	1.8217	1.7684	1.7110
26	4.2252	3.3690	2.9751	2.7426	2.5868	2.4741	2.3883	2.3205	2.2655	2.2197	2.1479	2.0716	1.9898	1.9464	1.9010	1.8533	1.8027	1.7488	1.6906
27	4.2100	3.3541	2.9604	2.7278	2.5719	2.4591	2.3732	2.3053	2.2501	2.2043	2.1323	2.0558	1.9736	1.9299	1.8842	1.8361	1.7851	1.7307	1.6717
28	4.1960	3.3404	2.9467	2.7141	2.5581	2.4453	2.3593	2.2913	2.2360	2.1900	2.1179	2.0411	1.9586	1.9147	1.8687	1.8203	1.7689	1.7138	1.6541
29	4.1830	3.3277	2.9340	2.7014	2.5454	2.4324	2.3463	2.2782	2.2229	2.1768	2.1045	2.0275	1.9446	1.9005	1.8543	1.8055	1.7537	1.6981	1.6377
30	4.1709	3.3158	2.9223	2.6896	2.5336	2.4205	2.3343	2.2662	2.2107	2.1646	2.0921	2.0148	1.9317	1.8874	1.8409	1.7918	1.7396	1.6835	1.6223
40	4.0848	3.2317	2.8387	2.6060	2.4495	2.3359	2.2490	2.1802	2.1240	2.0772	2.0035	1.9245	1.8389	1.7929	1.7444	1.6928	1.6373	1.5766	1.5089
60	4.0012	3.1504	2.7581	2.5252	2.3683	2.2540	2.1665	2.0970	2.0401	1.9926	1.9174	1.8364	1.7480	1.7001	1.6491	1.5943	1.5343	1.4673	1.3893
120	3.9201	3.0718	2.6802	2.4472	2.2900	2.1750	2.0867	2.0164	1.9588	1.9105	1.8337	1.7505	1.6587	1.6084	1.5543	1.4952	1.4290	1.3519	1.2539
∞	3.8415	2.9957	2.6049	2.3719	2.2141	2.0986	2.0096	1.9384	1.8799	1.8307	1.7522	1.6664	1.5705	1.5173	1.4591	1.3940	1.3180	1.2214	1.0000

Appendix III: The student's *t* distribution

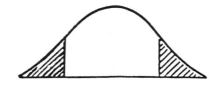

d.f.	0.9	0.8	0.7	0.6	0.5	0.4	Probability 0.3	0.2	0.1	0.05	0.02	0.01	0.001
1	0.158	0.325	0.510	0.727	1.000	1.376	1.963	3.078	6.314	12.706	31.821	63.657	636.619
2	0.142	0.289	0.445	0.617	0.816	1.061	1.386	1.886	2.920	4.303	6.965	9.965	31.598
3	0.137	0.277	0.424	0.584	0.765	0.978	1.250	1.638	2.353	3.182	4.541	5.841	12.924
4	0.134	0.271	0.414	0.569	0.741	0.941	1.190	1.533	2.132	2.776	3.747	4.604	8.610
5	0.132	0.267	0.408	0.559	0.727	0.920	1.156	1.476	2.015	2.571	3.365	4.032	6.869
6	0.131	0.265	0.404	0.553	0.718	0.906	1.134	1.440	1.943	2.447	3.143	3.707	5.959
7	0.130	0.263	0.402	0.549	0.711	0.896	1.119	1.415	1.895	2.365	2.998	3.499	5.408
8	0.130	0.262	0.399	0.546	0.706	0.889	1.108	1.397	1.860	2.306	2.896	3.355	5.041
9	0.129	0.261	0.398	0.543	0.703	0.883	1.100	1.383	1.833	2.262	2.821	3.250	4.781
10	0.129	0.260	0.397	0.542	0.700	0.879	1.093	1.372	1.812	2.228	2.764	3.169	4.587
11	0.129	0.260	0.396	0.540	0.697	0.876	1.088	1.363	1.796	2.201	2.718	3.106	4.437
12	0.128	0.259	0.395	0.539	0.695	0.873	1.083	1.356	1.782	2.179	2.681	3.055	4.318
13	0.128	0.259	0.394	0.838	0.694	0.870	1.079	1.350	1.771	2.160	2.650	3.012	4.221
14	0.128	0.258	0.393	0.537	0.692	0.868	1.076	1.345	1.761	2.145	2.624	2.977	4.140
15	0.128	0.258	0.393	0.536	0.691	0.866	1.074	1.341	1.753	2.131	2.602	2.947	4.073
16	0.128	0.258	0.392	0.535	0.690	0.865	1.071	1.337	1.746	2.120	2.583	2.921	4.015
17	0.128	0.257	0.392	0.534	0.689	.0863	1.069	1.333	1.740	2.110	2.567	2.898	3.965
18	0.127	0.257	0.392	0.534	0.688	0.862	1.067	1.330	1.734	2.101	2.552	2.878	3.922
19	0.127	0.257	0.391	0.533	0.688	0.861	1.066	1.328	1.729	2.093	2.539	2.861	3.883
20	0.127	0.257	0.391	0.533	0.687	0.860	1.064	1.325	1.725	2.086	2.528	2.845	3.850
21	0.127	0.257	0.391	0.532	0.686	0.859	1.063	1.323	1.721	2.080	2.518	2.831	3.819
22	0.127	0.256	0.390	0.532	0.686	0.858	1.061	1.321	1.717	2.074	2.508	2.819	3.792
23	0.127	0.256	0.390	0.532	0.685	0.858	1.060	1.319	1.714	2.069	2.500	2.807	3.767
24	0.127	0.256	0.390	0.531	0.685	0.857	1.059	1.318	1.711	2.064	2.492	2.797	3.745
25	0.127	0.256	0.390	0.531	0.684	0.856	1.058	1.316	1.708	2.060	2.485	2.787	3.725
26	0.127	0.256	0.390	0.531	0.684	0.856	1.058	1.315	1.706	2.056	2.479	2.779	3.707
27	0.127	0.256	0.389	0.531	0.684	0.855	1.057	1.314	1.703	2.052	2.473	2.771	3.690
28	0.127	0.256	0.389	0.530	0.683	0.855	1.056	1.313	1.701	2.048	2.467	2.763	3.674
29	0.127	0.256	0.389	0.530	0.683	0.854	1.055	1.311	1.699	2.045	2.462	2.756	3.659
30	0.127	0.256	0.389	0.530	0.683	0.854	1.055	1.310	1.697	2.042	2.457	2.750	3.646
40	0.126	0.255	0.388	0.529	0.681	0.851	1.050	1.303	1.684	2.021	2.423	2.704	3.551
60	0.126	0.254	0.387	0.527	0.679	0.848	1.046	1.296	1.671	2.000	2.390	2.660	3.460
120	0.126	0.254	0.386	0.526	0.677	0.845	1.041	1.289	1.658	1.980	2.358	2.617	3.373
∞	0.126	0.253	0.385	0.524	0.674	0.842	1.036	1.282	1.645	1.960	2.326	2.576	3.291

Index